MOTIVATIONAL INTERVIEWING
IN NUTRITION AND FITNESS

Applications of Motivational Interviewing

Stephen Rollnick, William R. Miller,
and Theresa B. Moyers, Series Editors

www.guilford.com/AMI

Since the publication of Miller and Rollnick's classic *Motivational Interviewing*, now in its third edition, MI has been widely adopted as a tool for facilitating change. This highly practical series includes general MI resources as well as books on specific clinical contexts, problems, and populations. Each volume presents powerful MI strategies that are grounded in research and illustrated with concrete "how-to-do-it" examples.

Motivational Interviewing in Health Care:
Helping Patients Change Behavior
Stephen Rollnick, William R. Miller, and Christopher C. Butler

Building Motivational Interviewing Skills: A Practitioner Workbook
David B. Rosengren

Motivational Interviewing with Adolescents and Young Adults
Sylvie Naar-King and Mariann Suarez

Motivational Interviewing in Social Work Practice
Melinda Hohman

Motivational Interviewing in the Treatment of Anxiety
Henny A. Westra

Motivational Interviewing, Third Edition: Helping People Change
William R. Miller and Stephen Rollnick

Motivational Interviewing in Groups
Christopher C. Wagner and Karen S. Ingersoll, with Contributors

Motivational Interviewing in the Treatment of Psychological Problems,
Second Edition
Hal Arkowitz, William R. Miller, and Stephen Rollnick, Editors

Motivational Interviewing in Diabetes Care
Marc P. Steinberg and William R. Miller

Motivational Interviewing in Nutrition and Fitness
Dawn Clifford and Laura Curtis

MOTIVATIONAL INTERVIEWING
in Nutrition and Fitness

DAWN CLIFFORD
LAURA CURTIS

*Series Editors' Note by Stephen Rollnick,
William R. Miller, and Theresa B. Moyers*

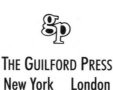

THE GUILFORD PRESS
New York   London

Library of Congress Cataloging-in-Publication Data

Names: Clifford, Dawn, author. | Curtis, Laura, author.
Title: Motivational interviewing in nutrition and fitness / Dawn Clifford,
    Laura Curtis.
Description: New York : The Guilford Press, [2016] | Series: Applications of
    motivational interviewing | Includes bibliographical references and index.
Identifiers: LCCN 2015042791| ISBN 9781462524181 (paperback : acid-free
    paper) | ISBN 9781462524198 (hardcover : acid-free paper)
Subjects: LCSH: Nutrition counseling. | Physical fitness. | Motivational
    interviewing. | Health promotion. | Psychotherapist and patient. | BISAC:
    MEDICAL / Nursing / Nutrition. | PSYCHOLOGY / Psychotherapy / Counseling.
    | MEDICAL / Sports Medicine.
Classification: LCC RM218.7 .C55 2016 | DDC 615.8/54—dc23
LC record available at http://lccn.loc.gov/2015042791

About the Authors

Dawn Clifford, PhD, RD, is Associate Professor and Director of the Didactic Program in Dietetics in the Department of Nutrition and Food Science at California State University, Chico. In addition, she cofounded and is currently Director of FitU, a peer mentoring nutrition and exercise counseling program on campus. She received the Outstanding Dietetics Educator Award from Nutrition and Dietetic Educators and Preceptors, a practice group of the Academy of Nutrition and Dietetics. Dr. Clifford conducts research and is an accomplished speaker in the areas of motivational interviewing and non-diet approaches to health and wellness. She has published several research articles in the *Journal of Nutrition Education and Behavior* and written curricula for *Today's Dietitian* and *Nutrition Dimensions*. She is a member of the Motivational Interviewing Network of Trainers (MINT).

Laura Curtis, MS, RD, is Director of Nutritional Services at Glenn Medical Center in Willows, California, where she provides clinical nutrition services to patients in acute care and is a nutrition therapist for the outpatient clinic. In addition, she serves as a preceptor to undergraduate dietetic students and is a part-time lecturer at California State University, Chico. Ms. Curtis has extensive training in motivational interviewing at both the undergraduate and graduate levels. As a nutrition therapist, she provides counseling to patients with conditions such as diabetes, heart disease, and disordered eating, and to those considering bariatric surgery. In her counseling, she pairs motivational interviewing with the non-diet principles of intuitive eating and Health at Every Size.

Series Editors' Note

Health care practitioners are under strain to "make the patient change" when it comes to eating right and exercising. Colleagues make referrals for behavior change counseling with certain goals in mind. As the recipient of the referral, it's easy to feel pressured into giving advice when your client so clearly needs to make lifestyle changes.

Motivational interviewing (MI) was developed to improve the conversation about behavior change. It started in the addictions field more than 30 years ago and was gradually refined, subjected to research scrutiny, and extended into other fields. This book provides a good example of this extension, since many of the challenges that arise in other fields converge on the subjects of eating and exercise: we can't make people change, only they can; reluctance to change is a widespread puzzle; and change itself is often not as simple as we would like it to be.

The authors of this book highlight and illustrate these themes from the first chapter to the last, and point to how practitioners might adjust their style and techniques to achieve outcomes that are more satisfying for all involved. The familiar exchanges about diet and exercise turn into something that is unique to each individual, allowing practitioners to develop their skills as they discover the motivations that drive the client.

Some of the shifts required to use MI well are quite radical. For example, one needs to view clients as people with strengths, not just as patients with a list full of pathologies. Empathic listening is key for not only keeping the conversation grounded in the individual, but also gently pointing the conversation in the direction of change, and paying attention to the client's language of change.

In one sense, this book is an invitation to change for practitioners themselves—changing the way they execute nutrition and fitness counseling. Using MI can involve far less strain and tension, in that you don't have to come up with all the answers yourself—that's the client's task. On the other hand, this invitation also involves a kind of listening and caring in the service of change that requires patience, curiosity, and thoughtfulness. The book shines with these qualities, and we welcome it with open arms into the series on applications of MI.

STEPHEN ROLLNICK, PhD
WILLIAM R. MILLER, PhD
THERESA B. MOYERS, PhD

Contents

PART IV. BEYOND THE BASICS

PART V. A CLOSER LOOK AT MOTIVATIONAL INTERVIEWING IN NUTRITION AND FITNESS INDUSTRIES

Purchasers of this book can download the handouts
from *www.guilford.com/clifford-forms*
for personal use or use with individual clients.

MOTIVATIONAL INTERVIEWING IN NUTRITION AND FITNESS

Introduction

Watch ice skating on television and notice how the skaters glide across the ice with ease and grace. Spins and jumps look effortless. Even on a bad day, their confidence on the ice and timing with the music are enough to bring fans to their feet in applause. It looks easy. Anyone who has stepped out onto the ice knows that without years of training, ice skating can be a painful experience. One wrong step on that smooth, slippery surface can bring you falling to your knees. It's a lot harder than it looks.

Similarly, you may be wondering about counseling in the nutrition and fitness fields. How hard can it be? Who *wouldn't* want to change their eating and exercise patterns for the better? Perhaps you made some changes yourself in these areas and are quite proud of your accomplishments. Possibly, you are a fan of healthy eating and being active. However, having healthy lifestyle patterns doesn't automatically make you an expert in counseling others to follow your lead.

Thanks to courageous efforts by public health educators, medical professionals, and even physical education teachers, we all by now know the importance of keeping our bodies healthy. We also know it's not easy to do, and that even despite a firm conviction to eat well and exercise, our motivation to do so waxes and wanes. One day you might wake up fueled by your intention to start eating more fruits and vegetables. You head to the store, buy a few different varieties, take them home, and incorporate them into your meals and snacks. The next day is a little busier, and you aren't able to get to the grocery store, so you end up eating a chocolate chip muffin from the vending machine in your office.

Clients are often ambivalent about change. Just as the definition of ambivalence states, clients frequently experience "simultaneous and contradictory attitudes or feelings" about changes regarding nutrition and exercise (*www.merriam-webster.com*). A young working mother wants to be fit and healthy so she can keep up with her children and be active in

1

their lives for years to come. However, when she leaves her children in the evening to go to the gym, she feels it takes away from their quality time as a family.

How would a nutrition or fitness professional help motivate this mother to incorporate regular physically activity into a busy and exhausting life? Would you give this mother a list of reasons to stay faithful to her gym routine? Would you warn her of the negative health outcomes if she doesn't? This *directive* style of counseling typically backfires, decreasing the likelihood of long-term change.

A client's motivation can be strongly influenced by a health professional's communication style. Imagine you were the working parent described above who is ambivalent about exercising regularly. How would you want your counselor to approach the topic? Choose from Counselor A or B below:

- Counselor A tells you what to do and then tries to convince you by telling you all the horrible things that might happen to you if you don't.

Or

- Counselor B listens to your concerns and desires, answers your questions, and is nonjudgmental and respectful.

Chances are good that you would prefer to work with Counselor B. As individuals, we like to be in charge of our own health decisions, and we feel most respected when we are heard and our feelings are considered.

MOTIVATIONAL INTERVIEWING BASICS

Motivational interviewing (MI) is "a collaborative, goal-oriented style of communication with particular attention to the language of change. It is designed to strengthen personal motivation for and commitment to a specific goal by eliciting and exploring the person's own reasons for change within an atmosphere of acceptance and compassion" (Miller & Rollnick, 2013, p. 29). William Miller and Stephen Rollnick developed MI and published their first book in 1992. While this client-centered counseling style has evolved over the last few decades, their third edition continues to represent MI as an empathetic listening style that supports clients in convincing themselves that they ought to change.

The primary goal of MI is to increase the client's interest in making a positive change through evoking his or her interest in the new behavior and disinterest in maintaining status quo. In MI, certain counseling techniques are used to encourage clients to explore and resolve ambivalence. In addition, the counselor helps the client see how a behavior change might align with future goals and values. Most important, an MI counselor nurtures the client's hope and confidence.

Clients typically know what they should do with regard to eating and physical activity, but there are many reasons why they don't. Counselors who use an MI style assume their clients are the experts. The client knows what works best, and the nutrition or fitness counselor is simply there to help the client figure it out.

As presented by Miller and Rollnick, a counselor who uses MI is like a guide dog for an individual with impaired vision. The person with the vision impairment knows where she would like to go. In the same way, a client seeking assistance in making health behavior changes knows which changes she would like to make. However, she needs a guide dog—the clinician—to help navigate the obstacles along the way.

In general, lecturing, confronting, coercing, or threatening the client doesn't work. In the same way, a guide dog is not going to pull his owner toward the post office if the owner *really* wants to go to the park. But the guide dog can walk alongside the owner and help her not fall into holes or run into poles.

This gentle guiding style used in MI puts the client in charge, promoting adherence to a specific behavior change. The client begins taking ownership of the behavior; it becomes the client's goal, not to please the counselor, but because it is important to the client.

Motivational interviewing is an exciting way of talking about change, which many researchers have demonstrated to be effective within the realm of nutrition and fitness (Armstrong, Mottershead, Ranksley, Sigal, & Campbell, 2011; Bean et al., 2015; Campbell et al., 2009; Christison et al., 2014; Neumark-Sztainer et al., 2010; Van Keulen et al., 2011; MacDonell, Brogan, Naar-King, Ellis, & Marshall, 2012; Miller et al., 2014).

However, MI isn't unique to nutrition and fitness. It has been used in a variety of disciplines for decades (Frey et al., 2011; Heckman, Egleston, & Hofmann, 2010; Lundahl et al., 2013; McMurran, 2009). The techniques are versatile to all behavior changes, be it ending or moderating drug and alcohol use, medication adherence, or dental care. In fact, MI has been touted as the all-purpose Swiss Army knife of behavior change counseling. However, it's not magic, and using MI with a client doesn't guarantee change. It simply increases the probability of change.

A LITTLE ABOUT THIS BOOK

This book is for students, interns, and professionals in a range of fields providing nutrition and fitness counseling. Whether you are new to this work or a seasoned professional, these pages include counseling strategies essential in helping clients make permanent changes in eating and activity.

Nutrition and fitness counseling is occurring in a variety of settings and continues to grow. Nutrition and fitness professionals must be armed with skills to encourage clients to adopt lasting changes. Practitioners in hospitals, health clinics, doctor's offices, summer camps, community programs, worksite wellness programs, private practices, and telehealth all benefit from learning how to motivate clients to improve eating and activity patterns.

Professionals such as registered dietitian nutritionists, clinicians, nurses, wellness or health coaches, community nutritionists, personal trainers and exercise counselors, PE teachers, and coaches spend their days talking to clients about healthy dietary and exercise changes. What happens to clients when they get home from their appointments? Do they put what they've learned into action? This book is for professionals who care about the success of their clients, not just the day, week, or month after their visits, but for years to come.

Health care practitioners may be wondering how MI fits in with the models, systems, and processes unique to each discipline. For example, in the field of nutrition and dietetics, the Nutrition Care Process (NCP) is the guiding model for providing evidence-based care (Lacey & Pritchett, 2003). The NCP consists of four steps: (1) assessment, (2) diagnosis, (3) intervention, and (4) monitoring/evaluation.

MI does not replace the NCP, but instead is incorporated into each step. Insights for melding MI and the NCP will be mentioned throughout the book. Other terms featured in nutrition and fitness settings like scope of practice (Academy Quality Management Committee & Scope of Practice Subcommittee of the Quality Management Committee, 2013a), mindful eating (Mathieu, 2009), and American College of Sports Medicine (ACSM) guidelines (Garber et al., 2011) will be addressed in light of MI, making this book a complete resource for practitioners who wish to improve their behavior change counseling skills.

In Part I of this book you will learn about the principles that make MI effective. In Part II we will take you step by step through a typical MI appointment in nutrition and fitness counseling, learning the various components of a session. Part II introduces the four processes within an MI session: (1) engaging the client, (2) inviting the client to focus on a topic, (3) evoking the client's feelings about change, and (4) assisting the client in the planning process of making the change. In this section, we will use scenarios and dialogue to demonstrate the four processes and specific communication techniques. It's one thing to read about a skill or technique, but it's much more fruitful to see it in action. We hope that these dialogues will help you apply these techniques in your own practice.

Part III includes information on specific MI communication techniques:

open-ended questions, reflections, affirmations, and summaries. These are known as the microskills of MI and are used throughout each appointment. When used correctly, these types of questions and statements can demonstrate empathy and help the client consider personal feelings regarding behavior change. In this section you will learn common evoking open-ended questions that are appropriate for nutrition and fitness counseling sessions. We'll also explain and demonstrate affirmations, reflections, and summaries. You will understand the importance of these skills in promoting client autonomy and moving him or her toward change.

Part IV will give new perspectives on topics that commonly arise in nutrition and fitness appointments. We'll address questions unique to nutrition and fitness counseling, such as: How do you dispel diet myths in a nonjudgmental manner? How do you promote realistic goal setting and help clients avoid setting short-lived New Year's resolutions? How do you promote fitness and health without leading clients to obsess about weight and appearance? Discussions of weight and health are so common in nutrition and fitness counseling that we devote an entire chapter to helping practitioners navigate this complicated topic with their clients.

The latest research on weight and health is resulting in a shift among practitioners away from weight-focused counseling toward what's called *weight-neutral counseling* (Ramos Salas, 2015; Tylka et al., 2014). Researchers are finding that diets, no matter which you use, don't work (Mann et al., 2007). Dieters lose weight at first, but almost always gain it back along with body insecurities, emotional ties to food, and a suppressed metabolism (MacLean, Bergoulgnan, Cornier, & Jackman, 2011; Neumark-Sztainer et al., 2006). Nutrition and fitness professionals who conduct weigh-ins, promote calorie counting, and assign miserable exercise regimens will soon be a distant memory.

Nutrition and fitness counselors are inviting clients to focus on sustainable, more realistic eating and activity patterns, instead of fixating on the scale. By taking the focus off of weight loss and body composition, and instead concentrating on developing a positive relationship with food and exercise, clients can avoid the emotional roller coaster associated with the dieting mindset while improving overall health and wellness. This non-diet approach has been found to be effective in promoting health, especially emotional health, and is preferred by clients (Clifford et al., 2015; Schaefer & Magnuson, 2014).

Sample MI dialogues throughout the book will remain consistent with this weight-neutral, non-diet approach, and include concepts such as mindful eating and discovering joyful physical activity patterns.

While it's entirely possible to use MI techniques in weight-focused counseling, the risk of doing so includes a vicious cycle of yo-yo dieting, disordered eating patterns, and body dissatisfaction. We believe MI and non-diet approaches make a beautiful marriage. Both involve exploring the client's personal thoughts and feelings about change and promote a non-judgmental self-exploration.

Food and feelings can be complex. Food, activity, and dieting can be used as coping tools for negative emotions, making behavior change counseling challenging at times. It can be a relief to remember that nutrition and fitness professionals are part of a client's health care team and can be the first to identify when a client might benefit from additional services. See more about making referrals to the appropriate health care professionals in Appendix 1, "Making Referrals," located at the end of this book.

Within one's scope of practice, a nutrition and fitness counselor using MI encourages a client to become curious about barriers to change, emotional ties to food and exercise, triggers for overeating, and roots of body image and self-esteem. MI is the perfect vehicle for inviting clients to explore how their nutrition and fitness patterns relate to other areas of wellness. Counselors who are able to bridge the gap between nutrition, exercise, and motivation will find they are better equipped to help clients actually reach and maintain their health goals.

Not everyone *wants* to change. However, through the use of strategic counseling techniques, unmotivated clients can become motivated—at times, even overnight. Mastering client-centered counseling techniques, on the other hand, does not happen overnight. The information provided in this book will give you tools and techniques to assist your clients and patients in making lifelong dietary and fitness changes. Combine this book with training and practice, and soon you'll be gliding across the ice with rhythm and grace.

PART I

Motivational Interviewing Basics

CHAPTER 1

The Complexities of Lifestyle Changes

The first step towards getting somewhere is to decide that
you are not going to stay where you are.
—UNKNOWN

Changing a behavior isn't easy. While clients have great intentions, they often struggle with consistent follow-through. They have grand hopes and dreams of taking care of their bodies, but then life gets in the way. Whether it's a new baby, a worrisome diagnosis, a job change, an unsupportive spouse, a flaky workout buddy, an unrelenting work schedule, or a vacation, the joys and challenges of life take us off course on the winding road toward health.

Before we can spell out the best strategies for assisting others in making permanent lifestyle changes, it's important to take a moment and discuss the complexities of change. In order to develop empathy for clients, it's often helpful to consider your own health patterns. Think about positive behaviors that you do naturally without any prompting. For many, brushing teeth twice a day is an ingrained habit. For the regular teeth brushers, how did it become so easy? Why do you do it? It's likely because the benefits of the behavior outweigh the costs. Taking a few minutes in the morning and the evening to brush your teeth gives you fresher breath and fewer cavities. Fresh breath improves your social life, and having fewer cavities lowers your dental bills. Taking care of your teeth may reduce oral pain, enhance your smile, and reduce your chance of losing teeth as you age. For regular brushers, the cost of a few minutes each day is worth the benefits of healthy teeth and gums.

Now consider a health behavior change that you've wanted to make but haven't quite attempted. What's keeping you from making that change? Perhaps you've been meaning to start flossing your teeth. You know the benefits of flossing your teeth, and your dental hygienist recommended that you floss daily, but you haven't started. The cost of flossing is a little higher than the cost of brushing your teeth: it tacks on a few extra minutes to your teeth-brushing regimen. Plus you may have to put up with bleeding and sore gums at first. While the benefits are similar to brushing, you may not be convinced it's necessary to maintain dental health. If you aren't currently flossing regularly, it's likely you don't think the benefits outweigh the costs, or maybe you haven't given it much thought. What would motivate you to make that change? Consider this question as we explore the complexities of making a behavior change.

STAGES OF CHANGE

Prochaska and DiClemente hypothesized that there are different stages of change (Prochaska & DiClemente, 1984). A person doesn't typically wake up one day, decide to change a behavior and then successfully maintain that change until the day he dies. Typically, an individual moves through stages. These stages of change are part of a behavior change theory known as the transtheoretical model (TTM).

While the TTM was developed around the same time as MI, they are quite distinct. TTM is a theory, whereas MI was developed from within practice; it is not a theory but a style and method for assisting others to make changes (Miller & Rose, 2009). However, it's useful to understand the stages of change that your clients experience in order to more fully grasp and appreciate the efficacy of MI.

There are five stages of change presented by the TTM: precontemplation, contemplation, preparation, action, and maintenance. Each stage is characteristic of certain thought patterns and behaviors.

1. *Precontemplation.* An individual in the precontemplation stage is either unaware or in denial that a change is necessary or warranted. In the nutrition and fitness counseling world, a client in precontemplation may open an appointment with, "I'm just here because my doctor made me come. Please don't take away my favorite foods. I've given up smoking and booze, and food is my last vice. You're going to take it away from me, aren't you?"

2. *Contemplation.* An individual in the contemplation stage is aware that a change needs to be made, but has mixed feelings about making the change. A client in this stage of change might say something like, "I probably shouldn't eat out every day for lunch, but I just get lazy in the morning and I'm always running late, so I hardly ever pack a lunch." The client has no plans to change and is on the fence about whether doing so would be worth the effort.

3. *Preparation.* In the preparation stage, the client is expressing a desire to make a behavior change within the next month and is seriously considering how he or she might go about doing so. A client in the preparation stage of change may state, "I know when I do try to eat more fruits and vegetables, I will need to go to the store more often so that I have fresh produce on hand."

4. *Action.* The action stage is most notably the hardest stage; in most cases it requires the client to expend physical energy. The stages before this one requires the client to expend mental energy, but the action stage is where the client actively makes the change he or she has been preparing for. A client in the action stage of change might say, "My doctor told me about my cholesterol last week, so I switched from butter to that fish oil margarine. It doesn't taste half bad."

5. *Maintenance.* Once the client has made the change consistently for 6 months, according to Prochaska and DiClemente, the client is in the maintenance stage of change. Clients who make it to the maintenance stage of change are still at risk for reverting to old patterns. However, the likelihood of maintaining the change is higher now that the change has become a regular part of the client's life for a significant amount of time. A client in the maintenance stage of change might say, "I've been riding my bike to work ever since I got out of cardiac rehab 2 years ago."

Now and then an individual may move linearly through the stages of change. What's more common, however, is for people to jump back and forth among the stages. Even within a single counseling session, a client might move from precontemplation all the way to preparation and back down to contemplation. The following narrative demonstrates the fluidity of the stages of change.

Jamie is a college student who decides she'd like to start adding 20 minutes of strength training twice a week to her busy schedule that includes work, school, and an active social life. She never gave strength training much thought (precontemplation) until she met her boyfriend, who enjoys lifting weights. He's an exercise science major and told her about how lifting weights can help improve muscle tone, bone strength, and posture. Jamie's mom always tells her that she slouches, so she likes the idea that doing strength training exercise might help. As she considers the change (contemplation) she wonders how she will fit it into her schedule and how she will learn the exercises. She doesn't have money for a personal trainer.

One summer, she discovers that her friend lifts weights a few times a week and asks her to demonstrate how to use the machines at the gym. Her friend agrees and they set a date for the next week (preparation). Jamie catches on quickly and figures out how to squeeze the time into her schedule by shortening the amount of time she spends on the cardio machines (action).

However, after the first week she is very sore and so decides to take a week off to recover (preparation). After the week is over, she goes on a summer vacation with her family. She restarts her routine 2 weeks later and lifts weights 2 days a week for the first 3 weeks of the fall semester (action). Then midterms hit and she isn't able to fit her gym routine into her schedule again until the spring semester (contemplation).

Jamie's spring semester is a little lighter, so she starts going to the gym again consistently for the spring semester and throughout summer (maintenance).

Sounds pretty normal, doesn't it? Behavior change often involves trial and error where consistency becomes an elusive goal. The term *ambivalence* is often used for this indecisive state of being. As a nutrition and fitness practitioner, it's important to learn how to recognize ambivalence and assist clients as they wade through the muddy waters of behavior change.

AMBIVALENCE 101

An individual who is in contemplation or preparation stages of change is in a state of ambivalence, experiencing mixed feelings about starting something new. It's almost as if his brain is split in two. Part of him wants to make the change and part of him doesn't.

Needless to say, the brain isn't so easily compartmentalized. In fact, the study of how the brain works and changes is an incredible science. Scientists seem to be learning more and more about *neural plasticity*, or the physical changes that occur in our neural circuitry based on our experiences. Consider the teeth brushing and flossing example. When you deviate from your old habits and start to do something new on a consistent basis, such as flossing your teeth, you are essentially growing new neural connections and pruning the old ones back. When you've entered into a state of maintenance with this behavior you've strengthened these new neural connections, making it easier to continue the behavior.

Understanding the concept of neural plasticity may help you understand why some habits are so hard to break. In its most basic form, a habit is just a particular pattern of neural connections. However, connections made over a long period of time or during a significant trauma will be more entrenched than others. At first, it can be uncomfortable to maintain a change, not because it is particularly hard to do, but because you are rewiring your brain. New behavior takes more mental energy and attention, whereas the old habit has become automatic. Ambivalence may simply be rooted in the decision to do something uncomfortable or unfamiliar. Falling back into old habits is often a welcomed comfort when change becomes unnerving or mentally taxing.

Ever-changing neural connections make the process of change a work in progress. A person can ebb and flow through the stages of change before their new behavior takes on any sense of permanence. A person experiencing ambivalence thinks change sounds good, but still has some reservations. He or she may start voicing reasons to make a change, but not make any commitments. Feeling two opposing ways about a behavior change is a normal part of the change process. It isn't something to avoid, but something to embrace, contemplate, and move through with your clients.

Feeling two opposing ways about a behavior change is a normal part of the change process.

In the following example, a middle-aged woman with newly diagnosed diabetes expresses mixed feelings about eating breakfast after years of skipping the morning meal.

"I stopped eating breakfast in high school. I was never hungry, and I always thought it would help me control my weight. Not that it really helped. My weight has been up, down, and all around. Now my doctor is putting me on medication and says if I don't eat, I could pass out. I'm just not hungry in the morning; it makes me feel sick just thinking about it. I hope I don't pass out and end up back in the hospital."

This next example highlights a man's ambivalence toward joining a tennis club after recovering from injuries he sustained during a severe car accident.

"I know I've got to get back into a regular exercise routine if I want to gain back my full function. My physical therapist says I'm ready, but I just don't know now. I guess I don't want to push myself. There's a lot of stuff I just can't do. But I know if I don't do anything, it will just get worse."

Spending time with ambivalence tends to help a client move through it. People tend to avoid it because it can be frustrating and uncomfortable to focus on conflicting priorities without making a decision. As a guide, you can shine a light on your client's ambivalence. When you home in on the ambivalence in a nonjudgmental way, your client can acknowledge the discrepancy, free from pressure. If ready to make a change, your client may want to start discussing strategies to adapt the change into everyday life.

Listening for Ambivalence: The Heart of MI

When listening for ambivalence, you will begin to hear client remarks both in favor of and opposed to making a behavior change. Comments made by the client that support change are known as *change talk*. Change talk sounds like this:

> "I don't want to end up on dialysis like my grandmother."
> "My friend has had a lot of success by switching out her soda for water. I might talk to her and try it out myself."
> "I'm tired of feeling sluggish. I can't believe how out of breath I get when I walk up a set of stairs."

Comments made by the client that support status quo are known as *sustain talk*. Sustain talk sounds like this:

> "The last diet I went on sent me to the poorhouse. I don't have the money to eat like that now that I'm retired."
> "There's no way I can eat in the morning. I hardly make it to work on time as it is."
> "By the time I get home, I'm exhausted. I can't imagine going to work out."

Often clients will speak change talk and sustain talk within the same sentence or dialogue. Ambivalence sounds like this:

> "I know I'd save money if I cooked more meals at home, but I hate doing dishes and cleaning the kitchen. When all is said and done, it's easier just to get takeout."
> "It wouldn't kill me to wake up a few minutes earlier, as long as I remember not to hit snooze too many times. Sometimes on cold mornings, I just can't help it."
> "I went for a walk the other day, but it was hot and humid. I did feel better after I went, but man, I hate this time of year."
> "I'd really like to learn how to play tennis, but I might make a fool of myself."

A good listener tunes his ears to his client's change talk and sustain talk. Change talk often predicts actual behavior change. Therefore, the practitioner elicits and highlights change talk throughout the MI session. This attribute of MI is a common thread revisited throughout this book.

The Root of Ambivalence

Ambivalence is often rooted in a discrepancy between an individual's values and actions. A client might value health and fitness, but think there is insufficient time to be more physically active. This results in a mismatch between where the client is and where the client wants to be. As the practitioner, part of your job is to help your client see that current patterns conflict with his or her values or health goals. In MI, you do this with great care using a curious, nonjudgmental stance, as in the script below:

> PRACTITIONER: You said you've wanted to try out a yoga class at your gym for a long time. What do you think is keeping you from going?
>
> CLIENT: I don't know, I'm probably just afraid to try something new. It will take me a while to get the hang of it, and I have to figure out if it's worth the risk of embarrassment.
>
> PRACTITIONER: You're concerned others might make certain judgments about your ability to do yoga.
>
> CLIENT: Yes, I hate to admit it, but it's true.
>
> PRACTITIONER: And yet you keep putting that on your to-do list.
>
> CLIENT: I want to be healthy, for one. Plus, my friends talk about yoga all the time. I want to feel like I can join in on their conversation. And I have really challenging teenagers who are pushing my buttons lately. I know I could use a way to de-stress.
>
> PRACTITIONER: You value your health and recognize that managing stress is an important way to stay healthy. Yoga has been a personal goal and interest for a long time now, and you're hesitant to get started. You sound pretty confident that if you got over some of your fears of surviving the first class, yoga would benefit you in a lot of ways. What do you think you will do?
>
> CLIENT: Yes, I know if I just did one or two classes, I'd be fine. I think if I make sure I go to my first class with one of my friends, I won't be as worried about the other people in the room.

Motivation for change is likely to increase when the client recognizes there is a discrepancy between a current choice and a personal goal. In the example above, the client is choosing to not attend the yoga class despite an interest in doing so. The practitioner uses reflective listening to help the client see this discrepancy, while giving the client full autonomy to attend the yoga class or not attend the yoga class.

> *Motivation for change is likely to increase when the client recognizes there is a discrepancy between a current choice and a personal goal.*

There were several examples of change talk in this brief dialogue, including "I want to be healthy," "I want to feel like I can join in on their conversation," and "I could use a way to de-stress." In short, MI techniques highlight for clients where they are and where they hope to be.

AMBIVALENCE IN DISGUISE: WHEN YOUR CLIENT WANTS THE QUICK FIX

There will be times when your client may not sound ambivalent. In fact, she may even sound excited and eager to change. However, her desire may be short lived. What happens in a few days, weeks, or months when she no longer feels like her changes are "working"? Year after year, millions of Americans make New Year's resolutions. However, only an estimated 40–46% of those who commit to a New Year's resolution are successful at maintaining the change 6 months later (Norcross, Mrykalo, & Blagys, 2002).

Given the high failure of self-change, it's hard to explain why people make resolutions. Perhaps it's the anticipation of the improved health or the psychological impact such as a boost of pride or confidence. Some researchers believe individuals like to attempt behavior changes because it gives them a feeling of control even if it doesn't work out in the end (Polivy & Herman, 1999, 2000).

Many turn to dieting in an effort to control food and weight when other areas of life are feeling out of control. Most overestimate the degree of control they have over their size and shape, ignoring the genetic determinants. It's easy to be lured in by images of thin or muscular bodies seen in the media, and consequently set unrealistic expectations and goals for their own weight and shape.

At the beginning of the New Year, clients believe the change they desire is easy to achieve, and their motivation is high. What is the result of setting unrealistic expectations for a behavior change? Goals are not met and clients become frustrated, discouraged, and they often throw in the towel. The phenomenon of attempting a behavior change with high hopes of successful outcomes has been called the false-hope syndrome (Polivy & Herman, 1999, 2000).

False-hope syndrome is a matter of overconfidence. It's hard not to feel overconfident when diet programs, in an effort to sell products, play into people's fantasies that they can change easily and see results quickly. Positive outcomes are routinely promised without any scientific evidence to support long-term success. Dieting researchers Herman and Polivy found that those who attempted to make a change and failed reported feeling worse about themselves and saw themselves as failures (Polivy & Herman, 1999).

Often clients attempt extreme dieting measures with the intention of changing temporarily for a big event such as a wedding, class reunion, or beach vacation. In a research study on brides and bridesmaids, 53% planned to lose weight for their weddings and 40% planned to do so through dieting (Prichard & Tiggemann, 2008).

What does this mean for nutrition and fitness practitioners? First, your client may not express any ambivalence, but that does not necessarily mean that he will succeed at making and sustaining a behavior change. Your client may seem eager to get started, and you immediately peg him as someone who is in the preparation stage of change. However, he may be looking for the quick fix or the magic bullet. At the infancy of a behavior change there can be excitement and curiosity, while the actual day-in and day-out efforts may become tedious and tiring. Furthermore, if the client has certain expectations in terms of outcomes or extrinsic reward, and those are not immediately noticed, he may lose steam.

A client who is a chronic yo-yo dieter may be excited to start another diet and anticipates immediate weight loss. However, if you're offering a non-diet approach that promotes taking the focus off of weight and onto health, you may receive some initial apprehension. In other words, the client may be in the preparation stage of change for starting another diet, but in the precontemplation stage of change for exploring a more realistic and balanced approach. She may be expecting an appointment filled with diet rules and lists of foods she's allowed to eat and foods she's not. Instead she gets evoking questions that invite her to explore emotions that drive eating and the etiology of her body image and binging behavior.

Clients often experience black-and-white thinking when it comes to nutrition and physical activity. Some experience rapid and extreme wavering back and forth from carefully counting calories and obsessively going to the gym to eating out all the time and snacking on sweets or salty foods at night to unwind. A client may state, "I'm good on the weekdays and then I let loose on the weekends." This all-or-nothing mentality sends clients on a vicious cycle starting with restricting favorite foods, skipping meals and snacks, or starting a tedious exercise regimen. Feelings of hunger and deprivation often lead to late-night treks to the kitchen (Polivy, Coleman, & Herman, 2005). Binges are followed by feelings of guilt and shame, which start the cycle over again, as clients go all in with a new diet scheme. This cycle has been described by many as the dieter's cycle, or the diet–binge cycle (Figure 1.1).

Presenting an Alternative Approach to the Quick-Fix Diet

How do you help clients recognize the emotionally exhausting consequences of dieting and replace this pattern with long-term solutions? Invite clients to share their stories, reflect on their dieting woes, and offer a new approach where lifestyle changes can be about variety, balance, and

Invite clients to share their stories, reflect on their dieting woes, and offer a new approach focused on variety, balance, and moderation, instead of restriction, avoidance, and desperation.

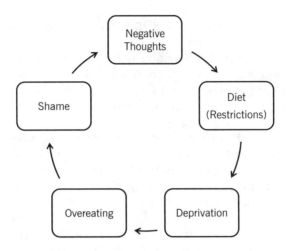

FIGURE 1.1. The diet–binge cycle. Copyright 2013 by Judith Matz, *judithmatz.com.* Reprinted by permission.

moderation, instead of restriction, avoidance, and desperation. Clients may not be expecting a gentle approach toward self-care, but often find that baby steps and self-compassion are the way to permanent change.

At times, the client's expectations for an appointment don't line up with the services offered. Most expect to meet with a nutritionist or dietitian and receive basic nutrition education. Most expect to meet with a fitness expert and receive a list of recommended exercises. Instead, MI puts the client in the driver's seat, where the client is encouraged to create his own list of changes and explore personal reasons for embarking on these new behaviors. This style takes the place of lecturing clients on why they need to change and how to do it. While nutrition and fitness education may still be part of the appointment, it often takes a back seat to what the client needs most—motivation to change. In the following dialogue, a client shares her struggles to maintain dietary restriction while the practitioner uses MI to highlight diet failures and change talk for a new approach to eating and activity.

> PRACTITIONER: What are you hoping to get out of our time together?
>
> CLIENT: I'm hoping you'll help me lose weight. I've dieted a number of times and I always gain it back. I'm hoping you have a diet for me that I can actually stick to.
>
> PRACTITIONER: You're tired of the emotional roller coaster that often goes with dieting and want to find more reasonable changes that you can stick to.

CLIENT: Yes. It would be nice if I lost a few pounds in the process, but I know as I get older, it's my health that I want to maintain.

PRACTITIONER: While it used to be more about appearances, today your primary motivation for seeing me is to get healthier.

CLIENT: Yes, exactly.

PRACTITIONER: Tell me a little more about your dieting experiences.

CLIENT: Well, I did the no-carb thing, and that worked for a little bit, but I started really missing bread with my cheese. I've also tried counting points or calories, and I'm good about keeping track of that for a little while and then it becomes more than my busy life can handle. I've tried the diets where you buy all the foods ahead of time, but that doesn't work for me now that I have a family.

PRACTITIONER: You've tried a number of diets and each one left you feeling deprived. What did you learn about yourself through those experiences?

CLIENT: I learned that I will never be a supermodel.

PRACTITIONER: You've changed your expectations and your definition of health.

CLIENT: Yes, I don't need to lose a lot of weight to be happy.

PRACTITIONER: It sounds like you'd like your weight to take a back seat to your focus on health, but at the same time, your happiness is still somewhat dependent on your size. Tell me more about that part.

CLIENT: Well, I guess that's true, though I don't like to admit it. I know when I was smaller, I felt better about myself. I liked the attention I would get from others whenever I lost weight. I felt like I was in really good shape and just had more energy in the day. I also liked that I could shop at the cute clothing stores. Now I do a lot of my shopping online. I used to love to shop.

PRACTITIONER: The high costs of cutting out foods you loved was worth it to you, at least in the short term, because of how being thinner made you feel.

CLIENT: Well, it was always worth it at first. But then it felt like my body became a sponge and every time I slipped up, my body would just absorb those calories and it seemed impossible to keep the weight off. And then as the weight would come back on, I'd start to feel embarrassed and wondered what people would think.

PRACTITIONER: It felt like an uphill battle with everyone watching.

CLIENT: Exactly! I'm sure they weren't watching, but they had to have noticed as my wardrobes would change with each new inch in my waist.

PRACTITIONER: It sounds like the ups and downs of dieting are what you truly hope to avoid. You want to learn to love and accept your body and at the same time discover ways to eat and exercise so that you feel fit, healthy, and energized. Would you be willing to explore these ideas a little more with me today?

CLIENT: Yes!

At the beginning of the dialogue, the client didn't sound ambivalent. She was set on her goal to lose weight. However, with some active listening and evoking questions from the practitioner, the client began to realize that what's most important to her is an overall feeling of health and fitness. She began to realize that previous attempts at the "quick fix" backfired and she became receptive to taking a different approach toward adopting more sustainable lifestyle changes.

FROM AMBIVALENCE TO ACTION: THE PRACTITIONER'S ROLE

Ambivalence is a fork in the road. Will the client choose to make the change, or keep things the same? The direction your client takes depends mostly on your style and guidance as the practitioner. In a state of ambivalence your client becomes conflicted and may feel a little embarrassed about having this discrepancy pointed out. In this delicate state of mind, she or he becomes highly responsive to the practitioner's communication style. A misstep can throw your client into a reactive stance and voicing *sustain talk*, that is, talk that favors the status quo. In the excerpt below, the client voices ambivalence about meal planning and preparation. The practitioner responds by trying to identify and fix the problem. Notice how this response leads the client to argue for the status quo. In doing this, the practitioner has essentially blocked the client from considering the change.

CLIENT: I hate cooking and especially doing dishes. I definitely do not have time for that. Plus, I'm a terrible cook. But I'm really tired of eating out all the time and it's so expensive.

PRACTITIONER: [*not* using MI] You need to make time. This is important.

CLIENT: I know, but we don't get finished with dinner until 8 o'clock already.

A misstep like the one above can easily derail a client's movement toward change. There are key strategies that you can use to help your clients move through ambivalence using a gentle, guiding manner. These strategies are dispersed throughout this book, but below is a glimpse of the most important factors in a practitioner's communication style that directly influence client ambivalence.

Taming the Righting Reflex

Most likely, you got into this line of work because you wanted to help people live healthier and happier lives. You are probably the type of person who cares for the people around you and wants to help others. This is a wonderful quality and one that makes you an empathetic and understanding practitioner. You also have an understanding of complex health topics that many people do not, and you're probably eager to share that knowledge with others. Our first inclination as nutrition and fitness practitioners when we hear a client's ambivalence is to start to nudge him or her forward by throwing out simple strategies for change. Does this sound familiar?

> CLIENT: I get home after work and I'm exhausted. I know I need to take a walk around the block, but it takes all of my energy just to get out of my work clothes and start making dinner.
>
> PRACTITIONER: [*not* using MI] What if you stopped at the gym before getting home? Sometimes you have to change your routine a little and you find that you have more energy.
>
> CLIENT: Maybe. I don't know. It's so crowded right after work.

Here's another example of a nutrition counselor reacting to ambivalence by giving unsolicited advice.

> CLIENT: My main problem is my snacking. My girlfriends and I get together twice a week to play cards and that's where I do a lot of my snacking. There's always a bowl of candy on the table while we play. I wouldn't eat it if it weren't right in front of me the whole time. They should know better than to serve that kind of stuff. Half of us are diabetic.
>
> PRACTITIONER: [*not* using MI] What if you brought your own snack? Here's a list of diabetic snacks that are quick and easy; perfect for a card table.
>
> CLIENT: Oh, I don't think so. You don't get between these ladies and their sweets.

As experts in nutrition and fitness, it can be difficult to restrain yourself from giving unsolicited advice when you see your clients struggling with ambivalence. This type of advice giving is also known as the *righting reflex*. The following sentence starters are all predictors that you're about to use the righting reflex.

"Why don't you just . . . ?"
"Hey, what about trying . . . ?"
"What you need to do is. . . . "

The righting reflex reflects a directive counseling style that includes giving advice or tips without gaining permission from the client. In the process of change, unsolicited advice becomes a roadblock that can interfere with the client's progression toward change. When a roadblock goes up, the client has to take a detour and think about how to respond to your advice, taking the focus off of strategizing a change. Use of the righting reflex may even stall out the client–practitioner relationship before it has a chance to get going. Although you have the best intentions, the way you go about giving advice and offering information is as important, if not more important, than the information itself.

People often consider the advice or recommendations of those they respect and trust. Using MI techniques helps you to gain respect and trust from your clients by treating them with unconditional positive regard, a concept first pioneered by the psychologist Carl Rogers (Rogers, 1995). Rogers believed that people have the resources within to bring about personal growth. By adopting an attitude of unconditional positivity toward people trying to change, you allow them the support they need to take responsibility for their behaviors and accept themselves as they are.

> *By adopting an attitude of unconditional positivity toward people trying to change, you allow them the support they need to take responsibility for their behaviors and accept themselves as they are.*

Putting the Client in the Driver's Seat

The righting reflex is just one way practitioners may inadvertently increase sustain talk when a client is ambivalent about change. An underlying power struggle often results when you use a directive communication style. At the end of the day, people end up doing what *they* choose to do. By honoring the client's control, or *autonomy*, you can avoid a power struggle and your counseling appointments will be more productive. This isn't to say that the client leads and you follow. MI is a guiding technique; you come alongside the client as a knowledgeable aide in the behavior change process. Honoring your client's autonomy tells him that he's in charge and you respect him from the minute he walks through the door. Defensiveness often melts away as your client feels supported.

Trying On the Client's Shoes

You won't always be able to relate to your client's experiences; it's generally impossible to actually walk a mile in another person's shoes. However, a key factor in assisting your client in navigating the maze of ambivalence is empathy. Empathy is defined as "the feeling that you understand and share another person's experiences and emotions" (*www.merriam-webster.com/dictionary/empathy*). Note that empathy does not involve you *actually going through another person's experiences and emotions* but instead *feeling that you understand* the experiences and emotions.

Empathy is essential in cultivating healthy human relationships. The key to developing empathy is being a good listener. Plus it takes a little bit of curiosity and imagination to understand what the client may be going through. It's normal to have mixed feelings about change. That's why it's important to set aside your personal agenda and attempt to understand your client's feelings of internal conflict.

Below are two dialogues. In the first, you can see the result of a counseling session in which the cardiac rehabilitation dietitian seems to lack empathy. In the second, you will notice the power of empathy in moving the client forward along the stages of change. Practitioner statements that directly express empathy are italicized.

Scenario 1

PRACTITIONER: Welcome to cardiac rehab. I'm the dietitian here and I see on your chart that you had a heart attack 3 weeks ago.

CLIENT: Yes, that's right.

PRACTITIONER: What questions do you have about what you should be eating?

CLIENT: I think I'm supposed to be watching how much fat I eat, right? My wife stopped cooking with butter years ago, so that won't be a problem.

PRACTITIONER: It's not just about what you need to cut out. It's also about what's missing. You'll also want to add foods like fruits, vegetables, legumes, and nuts, as well as be more physically active. Here, I have this handout for you to take home that explains more about these topics. I suggest you show this to your wife when you get home.

CLIENT: OK.

Scenario 2

PRACTITIONER: Welcome to cardiac rehab. I'm the dietitian here and I see on your chart that you had a heart attack 3 weeks ago. *That must have been really scary.*

CLIENT: Yes, it really freaked me out. I feel pretty lucky that we caught it early enough.

PRACTITIONER: You are relieved to have come through it all. I know you met with a dietitian briefly while you were in the hospital. Have any questions come up for you since then? *I know it can be overwhelming in the hospital when you're interacting with so many different people.*

CLIENT: Yes, my hospital stay was a whirlwind. And I only remember about half of it. It hasn't been too hard. We hadn't been cooking with butter for years, so we didn't really need to make any major changes.

PRACTITIONER: *Glad to hear it hasn't been too challenging.* I have a list of different topics here that we could discuss today, if you're interested. Are there any topics here that you'd like to go over?

CLIENT: Yes, we should probably talk about eating more fruits and vegetables. I'm sure there's more we could be doing there.

PRACTITIONER: Great. Let's do that. I have a list here of some ways to add more fruits and vegetables to meals and snacks, which you can take home to your wife, if you think she'd be interested, but first, tell me what you've already tried.

In the second scenario, the dietitian displays empathy and provides the client with a sense of autonomy. The client is in the driver's seat and the practitioner is demonstrating a desire to understand the client's perspective. The second scenario is slightly longer; it may take a little more time and patience in your interactions with clients to express these attributes. However, the payoff is extraordinary, as the client is much more likely to attempt and maintain a behavior change with this approach and return for follow-up visits.

Clients struggle when making changes to their eating and physical activity habits for a variety of reasons. In this chapter we've only scratched the surface of the complexities of behavior change. These useful techniques for assisting clients through ambivalence are revisited in great detail throughout the remaining chapters.

It is common to witness clients adopting unrealistic expectations for themselves, thinking they must do it perfectly or not at all. At times, they will get stuck, favoring to sustain the status quo until faced with significant negative outcomes.

As the practitioner, your communication style significantly influences your clients' decisions to make and maintain lifestyle changes. You not only influence *what* they decide to change but also *if* they will decide to change. By identifying ambivalence and helping your clients consider the discrepancies between their actions and values in a nonjudgmental and empathetic manner, they can successfully move forward through ambivalence and eventually achieve their health goals.

CHAPTER 2

The Spirit of Motivational Interviewing

People don't care how much you know until they know
how much you care.
—JOHN HANLEY

Doing motivational interviewing with someone is like
entering their home. One should enter with respect,
interest, and kindness, affirm what is good, and refrain
from providing unsolicited advice about how to arrange
the furniture.
—KAMILLA VENNER

As a practitioner, you will not physically be with your clients when they act
on health decisions. You won't be there when they are at the grocery store
or when they get off work and decide whether or not to go for that walk
you talked about. You, in effect, have absolutely no control over your clients' behaviors. They have the right to make decisions that do not support
their health. What they need from you is not a wagging finger or a repri-
mand; they need to be affirmed of their positive potential. Understanding
this will help you to take your rightful place in the counseling relationship,
not as a judge of their behavior, but as a guide to help them reach their
health goals. This chapter describes the most fundamental component of
MI: your mindset.

The mindset or underlying spirit of MI affects every aspect of how
you interact with a client, including verbal and nonverbal communication.
Miller and Rollnick (2013) have framed the spirit of MI using four key
concepts: partnership, acceptance, compassion, and evocation, which are
summarized in Figure 2.1.

Spirit of MI component	Definition	Examples of practitioner statements
Partnership	The practitioner functions as a partner or companion, collaborating with the client's own expertise.	"You'd like ideas for high protein foods. If you think it might help, we could make a list of protein-rich foods you already eat and then together we can brainstorm others you'd be interested in trying."
Acceptance	The practitioner communicates absolute worth, accurate empathy, affirmation, and autonomy support.	"You seem frustrated. On the one hand, you'd like to be more consistent about going to the gym, and, on the other hand, you don't enjoy working out on the fitness equipment there. There are times in your life when you've been very committed to going and you're realizing that the gym has lost its appeal. What do you think you'll do?"
Absolute worth	The practitioner emphasizes the inherent value and potential of every human being.	"I really appreciate you sharing how you feel about your body right now. These feelings are important, and I'm honored that you felt you could trust me with the information."
Accurate empathy	The practitioner perceives and reflects back the client's meaning.	"You hope that I'm going to give you information that will help you manage your blood sugars and at the same time, you're a little worried that you're going to have to give up certain foods that give you immense pleasure."
Autonomy	The practitioner accepts and confirms the client's irrevocable right to self-determination and choice.	"It's your body and you know yourself better than anyone else. Ultimately you get to decide which foods your body does best with."
Affirmation	The practitioner accentuates the positive, seeking and acknowledging a person's strengths and efforts.	"You are a fighter. You don't let anything stand in your way of accomplishing your goals."
Compassion	The practitioner acts benevolently to promote the client's welfare, giving priority to the client's needs.	"I am so sorry to hear that you and your family are going through this financial hardship. If you're interested, I'd be happy to provide you with some resources for obtaining free and reduced-priced meals in our community."
Evocation	The practitioner elicits the client's personal motivation for a particular change.	"How would making this change make your life better?"

FIGURE 2.1. The spirit of MI at a glance. Definitions based on Miller and Rollnick (2013).

PARTNERSHIP

In the "good old days" of nutrition and exercise counseling, the counselor acted as the expert and the client acted as the student. The nutrition or exercise expert would rattle off the different types of dietary and exercise changes that the client needed to make and the client would sit and listen.

Over the years, researchers have found flaws with this style of communication. Clients would brace themselves for the abuse, admit their faults right at the start, and sit expectantly for their punishment. For the majority, this style of counseling irritated and humiliated clients, resulting in high no-show rates and few follow-up appointments. A practitioner might even say, "I did *my* best, *he* was just unmotivated." William Miller, one of the founding fathers of MI, discovered that the counselor's communication style largely influences the outcome of a session. Perhaps it isn't that the client is unmotivated; the real issue is the counselor's communication style. Instead of writing off an unmotivated client, consider your role in evoking disinterest in behavior change.

In a consultation driven by MI, the practitioner avoids wearing the "expert hat" and instead comes alongside the client in a partnership role. Together, as a team, the practitioner and the client explore the client's world. The practitioner maintains an aura of curiosity as the client is guided to consider all angles of a behavior change. At times, tips may be provided, but they are offered if the client gets stuck and only with permission when the client is ready to change.

In an attempt to collaborate with the client, the practitioner might say, "It sounds like you're interested in packing a lunch more often to take to work, and that you'd like more ideas of foods you could pack. Would it be helpful to brainstorm together a list of packable lunch ideas?" By including the client in the process he is sure to leave your office with a list of foods he enjoys eating. Plus, he may feel more empowered to make the change because he played an active role in coming up with a solution.

The Expert Trap

In working *with* the client instead of *on* the client, the MI practitioner avoids falling into the expert trap. The *expert trap*, a term coined by Miller and Rollnick, occurs when a practitioner gives the impression that he has all the solutions to his clients' problems. Sometimes the practitioner can even come across as the "perfect eater" or "perfect exerciser" by describing solutions that have worked for him in the past. This can be problematic as it places the practitioner on a pedestal, making it hard to set a tone of partnership.

The expert trap occurs when imperatives are used. Imperatives are statements that express a command such as "You need to . . . " or "You should. . . ." These phrases suggest that the practitioner is the expert on what might work for the client. While it is true that the practitioner may have more knowledge on the topic of nutrition and fitness, the client knows what will work with her current lifestyle patterns. Furthermore, bringing attention to the knowledge and expertise of the practitioner diminishes the feeling of a partnership.

To enhance the spirit of collaboration, replace imperatives with "Some of my clients have found . . . What might work best for you?" For example, instead of, "You should check your blood sugars every morning," you can demonstrate a desire for partnership by replacing the imperative with, "My clients who check their blood sugars every morning find that they are more successful at keeping them in their goal range. What have you found?"

Figure 2.2 shows statements that represent the expert trap as well as alternative phrasing aimed to help create more of a partnership.

ACCEPTANCE

The practitioner brings an attitude of acceptance to the client–practitioner relationship. Acceptance, as described by the work of Carl Rogers, is multifaceted (Rogers, 1995). The practitioner conveys this attribute by communicating absolute worth, affirmation, autonomy, and accurate empathy.

Absolute Worth

Also known as unconditional positive regard, absolute worth is built on a foundation of basic trust. The client is inherently trustworthy and thus respected as an individual. According to Miller and Rollnick, and based on the ideas of Carl Rogers, "When . . . people experience being accepted as they are, they are freed to change" (Miller & Rollnick, 2013). In essence, the practitioner creates an optimal environment for the client to grow, supporting the client with genuine care and respect. "R-E-S-P-E-C-T" is not only a catchy tune, but can also serve as an acronym to help you communicate in a respectful way (Adapted from *www.budbilanich.com/r-e-s-p-e-c-t-dont-know-what-it-means-to-me*):

Recognize the inherent worth of all human beings.
Eliminate bias and stereotypes.
Speak *with* people, not at them.
Practice empathy.
Empower people to change.
Create an environment of trust.
Treat clients as the experts of themselves.

Practitioner response expressing the expert trap	Expert trap issue	Practitioner response expressing partnership	Partnership strategy
Client statement: "I know I don't eat enough fruit. I could probably do a better job in that area."			
"One way I like to get more fruits in my diet is by making fruit smoothies. I just add in some fruit, yogurt, and juice and blend it up."	Practitioner comes across as the "perfect eater" and does not first assess what types of changes interest the client.	"You'd like to eat more fresh fruit. What ideas to you have for adding more fruit? . . . Would you be interested in hearing one idea that's perfect for a hot day like today?"	Practitioner invites client to come up with her own ideas and then asks permission before providing the smoothie idea.
Client statement: "I'm looking for a new type of exercise that is more relaxing and easier on my joints. I've been under a lot of stress lately. Do you know of any?"			
"You should try yoga. It will make you stronger and help you manage your stress better."	Practitioner uses the imperative, "You should . . . "	"Some activities like yoga are geared toward stretching, strengthening, and relaxation. What are your feelings about those types of activities?"	Information is provided without imperatives. An open-ended question is used to assess client's interest.
Client statement: "My blood sugars have been a little higher than normal lately."			
"If you don't get your blood sugars under control, your kidneys are going to fail and I know you don't want to be on a kidney machine the rest of your life."	Practitioner threatens the client.	"You'd like to get your blood sugars down. What concerns you most about high blood sugars? [client responds] High blood sugars can negatively impact a couple of organs in the body. I'd be happy to share more about that, if you're interested."	Practitioner evokes concerns from the client, and then asks permission to share negative consequences.
Client statement: "I know I drink too much soda, but I hate the taste of diet drinks. I should try to drink more water, but it's really bland and boring. I need ideas for making water taste better."			
"I get bored with water too. And just like you, I don't like diet drinks. What I do is add a little bit of fruit juice to my water."	Practitioner comes across as the "perfect eater."	"Taste is important to you when selecting beverages. What ideas do you have for flavoring your water?"	Practitioner reflects what is important to the client and then asks client for ideas before providing others.

FIGURE 2.2. From expert trap to partnership. *(continued)*

Client statement: "I like your idea of adding more vegetables to the meals I already make. That shouldn't be too hard."			
"Yes, you could add vegetables to dishes like tacos, pastas, sandwiches, pizzas, and soups. Just sneak them into your meals."	Practitioner gives ideas without asking the client for ideas first and without asking permission.	"What ideas do you have for adding vegetables to the meals you already make? [client responds] Would you be interested in hearing some other meals that often taste great with added vegetables?"	Practitioner asks client for ideas first, then asks permission before sharing additional ideas.
Client statement: "I think I could fit in walks on the weekends, possibly one on Saturday and one on Sunday."			
"You're walking 2 days a week, which is a great start, but you want to aim for 5 days a week. Once you're exercising more often, you'll really start to notice a difference."	Practitioner sets client's goal without asking client first.	"Walking 2 days a week is a great start."	Practitioner honors what feels doable to the client.

FIGURE 2.2. (*continued*)

Practitioners view their clients through their own set of lenses that are shaped by their past experiences. Messages from friends, family members, and the media shape how we view others. Misshapen lenses result in disillusions or misconceptions like stereotyping, discrimination, and bias, all of which hinder the maturation of respect for the client.

Misshapen lenses result in disillusions or misconceptions like stereotyping, discrimination, and bias, all of which hinder the maturation of respect for the client.

Absolute worth is a key component of the spirit of MI as it emphasizes the importance of respecting all individuals, regardless of race, religion, socioeconomic status, sexual orientation, gender, or size. MI practitioners can cultivate a deep connection with clients when they clear their lenses and develop a genuine respect for all people. Clients respond positively when they feel cared for and accepted.

Accurate Empathy

A practitioner demonstrates accurate empathy when she takes an active interest in her client and attempts to understand her client's perspective.

Respecting Clients through
the Elimination of Weight Bias

One form of bias commonly seen in nutrition and exercise counseling is weight bias (Swift, Hanlon, El-Redy, Puhl, & Glazebrook, 2012; Campbell & Crawford, 2000). Health care professionals self-report bias and prejudice against overweight and obese patients. Obese patients report feeling stigmatized in health cares settings and are more likely to avoid routine preventative care (Amy, Aalborg, Lyons, & Keranen, 2006; Sikorski et al., 2011). Those experiencing stigmatization are more likely to suffer from depression and report feeling less motivated to adopt healthy lifestyle changes (Eisenberg, Neumark-Sztainer, & Story, 2003; Puhl & Brownell, 2006; Vartanian & Shaprow, 2008; Vartanian & Novak, 2011).

Nutrition and fitness professionals often believe people are responsible for their own weight and fail to lose weight because of poor self-discipline or a lack of willpower (Johnston, 2012). This belief system is unfounded and discounts the genetic component of body weight. It has been well researched that there are physiological mechanisms in place to counterbalance dieting efforts, making it nearly impossible for some people to lose weight and maintain weight loss (MacLean et al., 2011; Sumithran & Proietto, 2013). Some believe stigma and shame will motivate people to lose weight when, in fact, researchers have found the opposite to be true. Weight discrimination actually increases risk for obesity (Sutin & Terracciano, 2014).

The practitioner doesn't have to experience the same challenges in order to demonstrate empathy. She simply has to recognize and attempt to understand emotions that her client is experiencing.

Empathy is expressed in many ways in a counseling session through the use of both verbal and nonverbal communication. The practitioner shows empathy through a physical and calming presence, by inviting the client to share more about his or her experience, and through attentive and active listening.

Here are examples of counselor statements that demonstrate empathy:

"You feel anxious about your new diagnosis because you don't know how it will affect your future health status."

"When your mom gave you that look at the dinner table, how did it make you feel?"

"When your husband made that joke about your weight in front of your friends, it must have been really embarrassing."

"I can only imagine how hard it must have been to hear your husband say that."

Empathy isn't only communicated through words; facial expressions, body language, and tone of voice are also essential in demonstrating empathy. Any of the above statements could be phrased with a negative, condescending, mocking, or threatening tone, thereby failing to communicate genuine empathy. Therefore, demonstrating empathy involves the combination of a compassionate nonverbal communication style along with words that communicate a general interest and desire to understand the client.

Autonomy

We as humans hate to be told what to do. In fact, we often want to do exactly the opposite of what we are told we *should* do. What happens when clients are given complete freedom and respect to change or not change? They are often more open to change! When they don't feel pressured or coerced, they can openly choose what's best for them given what it is they value.

Comments that the practitioner may use to demonstrate client autonomy include:

> "Yeah, you could do that. How would that work for you?"
> "It's ultimately up to you to decide how to respond to the doctor's concern. What do you think you will do?"
> "That's one way to look at it. Would you be interested in hearing what other clients have tried?"
> "You are the expert of your body and you get to decide what works best for you."
> "Would you be interested in hearing some ideas that have worked for other clients? Some have tried using alternative transportation to work in order to gain more physical activity, others have tried using lunch breaks for activity, and others prefer doing more active things on the weekends. What do you think you will try?"

When imperatives such as "You should . . . " or "You have to . . . " are used, the client loses his or her sense of autonomy. While these terms sound harsh, practitioners often replace them with softer directive statements such as "What you'll want to do is . . . ," "What we're going to do is . . . ," or "The best way to . . . is. . . . " While these terms are less forceful, they can come across as very directive, crushing any hope for an autonomous client–practitioner relationship and robbing the client of the freedom of choice.

Let's say you are a client who is referred by a physician to see a nutritionist for "cholesterol lowering." Which of the following professionals would you rather see?

Nutritionist 1

"You mentioned your father had a heart attack when he was in his 50s. Given your family history of heart disease, it's really important that you make some significant changes in your eating habits. The last thing you want is to have a heart attack like your father. You're really going to need to watch your diet and get more exercise."

Nutritionist 2

"You mentioned your father had a heart attack when he was in his 50s. How does that piece influence your health patterns today? . . . You were referred here because of your elevated cholesterol. What was it like to receive that information? . . . What do you think you will do now? . . . How can I help? You're the expert of your life and body and you know what works best for you."

In the first scenario, the nutritionist tells the client that he should value his health and tries to pressure him to be more motivated to change. This excerpt also includes imperative language. In the second scenario, the nutritionist poses several questions. These questions help draw out the client's feelings related to a new diagnosis. In addition, through gentle questioning, the client is being asked to consider how he will respond to his new diagnosis. Client autonomy is enhanced when the client is asked what he plans to do instead of what he *should* do. Finally, the nutritionist asks the client how she can help. In doing so, she sends a message that the client is not alone in the predicament.

The client and nutritionist can collaborate to find viable solutions, should the client be interested in changing. In this second scenario, the nutritionist displays the spirit of MI through offering to collaborate, asking the client to consider how the new diagnosis fits in with his values and concerns, and giving the client autonomy to choose how he will respond.

Affirmation

Clients often have the skills and education required to start making changes. What they sometimes lack, however, is confidence in their ability to execute and sustain a specific behavior change. What clients need is a confidence boost. An MI practitioner best serves his clients when he acts as a hound dog, sniffing around for opportunities to affirm them.

Affirmations are statements regarding a client's positive attributes. Affirmations sprinkled throughout an MI session empower clients. At times, opportunities to affirm are obvious, and at other times they are subtle.

An experienced MI practitioner perks his ears to listen for opportunities to affirm. In doing so, he creates an environment where the client feels

> *An MI practitioner best serves his clients when he acts as a hound dog, sniffing around for opportunities to affirm them.*

respected, validated, and encouraged. In the following script, the practitioner affirms his client noticing both the obvious and more subtle client strengths.

> CLIENT: It's not that I can't cook. My girlfriend actually raves when I cook for her and her roommates. She even said that I should be on cooking shows after I made this Italian stuffed shells dish the other night. It's just that I hate doing dishes.
>
> PRACTITIONER: You've got some serious talent in the kitchen. [affirmation] You're also a good boyfriend and don't want to mess up your girlfriend's kitchen. [affirmation]
>
> CLIENT: Yeah, I guess I just need a magic cleaning wand.
>
> PRACTITIONER: Many of my clients are completely paralyzed in the kitchen when it comes to blending foods and flavors. You've got a leg up in this process since you have some skills. [affirmation] And even though you don't like cleaning, you don't always let that get in the way of treating your girlfriend to good food. [affirmation]
>
> CLIENT: Yes, that's true. I'm pretty lucky my mom taught me how to cook.

In this script the practitioner uses three affirmations, and in doing so, highlights the client's strengths in the behavior change process. Affirming the client demonstrates an overall appreciation and respect, further enhancing rapport with the client.

COMPASSION

> Be kind, for everyone you meet is fighting a harder battle.
> —PLATO

Compassion is an essential attribute of a nutrition and fitness practitioner. Compassion, altruism, and empathy are tightly linked but are not the same. There is often confusion surrounding these terms, as compassion often involves an empathic response and an altruistic behavior. Empathy refers to understanding and sharing feelings with another. Altruism is an action that benefits someone else but may not be a result of empathy or compassion. For example, a registered dietitian nutritionist may volunteer to give a speech to nutrition students, but the speaker may have an ulterior motive of promoting her private practice business.

Compassion involves genuine concern for the suffering of others, which is beneficial for physical and mental health and well-being. Researchers studying the psychology of happiness and human flourishing have found that connecting with others in a meaningful way helps people to enjoy better mental and physical health, ultimately speeding up recovery from disease (Diener & Seligman, 2004).

The practitioner conveys compassion through giving priority to the client's needs and by actively promoting the client's welfare. To remain a truly compassionate nutrition and fitness practitioner, consider the needs of your client. If the focus is on your self-gain, then it will be challenging to maintain an aura of compassion. For example, if the counselor must report a certain number of positive client outcomes to a supervisor, or talk a client into a certain number of sessions for profit, the appointment will quickly become self-focused instead of client focused.

> *The practitioner conveys compassion through giving priority to the client's needs and by actively promoting the client's welfare.*

Compassion is about seeking and valuing the well-being of others. The counseling techniques described in this book are not meant to provide means to manipulate clients to change. At the heart of motivational interviewing is the general desire to do all we can for our clients' well-being.

Maintaining compassion as a counselor can be a challenge at times. However, compassion fatigue occurs when we try to fix our clients. Clients voice many reasons why behavior change is hard. If we view these as excuses, then we may start to lose compassion for our clients. However, if we attempt to put ourselves in our clients' shoes and experience all of their life variables at play, we start to see that these aren't excuses, but genuine and valid barriers, concerns, and feelings.

Compassion fatigue occurs when the practitioner tries to control something he or she cannot control. A practitioner does have control over what he says and how he says it, but does not have control over the client's response. Compassion fatigue can be avoided through good self-care and focusing on the process of counseling and less so on the outcomes of counseling.

EVOCATION

Just as the term *motivational interviewing* implies, the counselor does do a great deal of interviewing to enhance motivation to change. The intent of the questioning is not to quiz or collect data from the client but to elicit or draw out certain feelings about a behavior change.

The practitioner is in some ways like a journalist. A journalist interviews experts in order to write a story. A good journalist is never the expert on the story. There's no way for a journalist to be an authority on every topic written. The journalist becomes informed on a topic only through researching it and interviewing individuals closest to the story. A journalist has to maintain an unbiased stance and an aura of curiosity. In addition, a journalist must use evocative questions to draw out the experiences, opinions, and emotions of his sources.

On the other hand, the intentions of the interviewing conducted by an MI practitioner are much different than those of a journalist. In journalism, the interviewing is for the journalist; in behavior change counseling, the interviewing is for the client. The interviewing is meant to prompt the client to talk about the behavior change. Motivation for change resides within the client. The practitioner elicits beliefs, feelings, ideas, and motivations from the client, often bringing the unconscious to the conscious mind. In doing so, the client is able to discuss the behavior change in relation to what she cares about.

Sure, we can tell clients why we think they should change. But would this motivate them to change? Not necessarily. In doing so, we may bring up reasons to change that they don't necessarily care about. Therefore it's most effective to elicit their personal reasons for change. Open-ended questions are best for encouraging clients to think about what's important to them and how it relates to their eating habits. Here are some examples of open-ended questions that may be used to evoke reasons to change from the client:

> "What possible long-term consequences of diabetes concern you the most?"
> "What motivated you to make this appointment?"
> "What concerns—if any—do you have about your eating habits?"
> "What are the reasons you'd like to make a change?"

Eliciting thoughts and feelings about change not only helps you to accurately highlight what is important to the client; it also helps the client to hear his true beliefs. Often, it's not until something is said aloud that a person really reflects on the validity of the statement. In that moment he is able to consider whether the belief represents a personal truth.

Eliciting thoughts and feelings about change not only helps you to accurately highlight what is important to the client; it also helps the client to hear his true beliefs.

For example, clients often complain about how big portion sizes are when they are served food at a restaurant. In many cases, this is because there is a common deeply held belief that one must eat everything on his or her plate and avoid any food waste. People then feel that large serving sizes are to blame for their overeating. Through some well-spoken questions, your client may come to the realization that she is needlessly overeating in order to fulfill a belief that no longer makes sense; she is eating in a way that harms her relationship with food. Used in this way, evoking is a powerful mechanism to help people understand and work through the beliefs and thoughts that have developed over time.

In Figure 2.3, the parents of a teenage girl struggling with bulimia take the first steps in getting eating disorder treatment. Observe how the practitioner uses affirmations, accurate empathy, compassion, partnership, and evocation to lay the groundwork for a client–counselor relationship built on respectful communication.

The spirit of MI requires the practitioner to make the extra effort to be fully engaged in the counseling process. At times, it is more challenging to be empathetic, systematically affirming and supporting the client's autonomy while going at his or her pace. Unfortunately, you can't run ahead past the finish line and look back yelling, "I know how you can do it! I get it! You just need to. . . . " The counseling style is more predictive of the client's motivation than the actual information you have to share.

Being committed to the spirit of MI will make you the type of practitioner who clients feel can understand and relate to them. By seeing yourself as a partner in your client's journey, you can focus on honing your skills of acceptance and compassion while evoking the very important and necessary details of your client's experience. It is from the spirit of MI that trust is laid down as a foundation for the motivation for change to take root and grow.

CLIENT: I'm so glad you're helping my daughter with her eating issues. It really freaked us out when we overheard her throwing up her food after her birthday celebration. We knew she was always self-conscious of her body, but we had no idea she was bulimic.	
PRACTITIONER: Your daughter is really fortunate to have parents who care and who knew to seek help.	*Affirmation*
CLIENT: Yes. The second we talked with her about it, we knew she was going to need help. We got on the phone to her doctor the next day.	
PRACTITIONER: You must have really been concerned. It can be very hard when someone you love is hurting. I'm glad you are here. For my younger clients, I like to meet with the parents separately at first since the support of family is so crucial in recovery.	*Accurate empathy* *Compassion*
CLIENT: Yes, we really want to help her and have no idea what to do.	
PRACTITIONER: You're stumped and you're hoping I have some answers for you. Perhaps we can put our heads together today and come up with a game plan.	*Partnership*
PRACTITIONER: You mentioned that Stephanie has always been self-conscious of her body. When did you start noticing her negative body image?	*Evocation*
CLIENT: Gosh, as early as second grade. I have a daughter in high school and she likes to read popular magazines. She'd leave them lying around the house and Melanie would pick them up and start asking me about different articles in there. Some of the articles had some shocking adult content, so I had to tell my older daughter to keep those in her room. But ever since then I could tell that Melanie started to see herself differently. She really looks up to my older daughter and I could tell she started comparing herself. I told her she had a great 8-year-old body and not to worry about it, but needless to say, that didn't do much.	
PRACTITIONER: Despite your best efforts to protect your daughter, she continues to be dissatisfied with her body.	*Affirmation*
CLIENT: Yes. It's like nothing I said mattered after that.	
PRACTITIONER: It's like your voice was lost in a sea of voices from the media. Sometimes we hope that a megaphone will do the trick.	*Compassion*
CLIENT: Yeah, that's right.	
PRACTITIONER: What else can you tell me about the messages your daughter ran into throughout her childhood about weight, food, and exercise?	*Evocation*

FIGURE 2.3. The spirit of MI alive in a counseling session. Notice the various components of the spirit of MI throughout this script excerpt.

PART II

The Four Processes
of Motivational Interviewing

CHAPTER 3

Engaging and Focusing

Attention is the rarest and purest form of generosity.
—SIMONE WEIL

MI is a bit of a dance. The dance of the MI counselor with the client flows gracefully and even seems to have rhythm to its steps. While the dance is not choreographed, there is structure and framing. As with ballroom dancing, there is a leader and follower. The counselor acts as the lead dancer, and provides gentle guidance across four distinct areas of the dance floor, known as the four processes of motivational interviewing:

1. Engaging
2. Focusing
3. Evoking
4. Planning

This chapter begins with an overview of the four processes and follows with details of the first two, engaging and focusing. The third and fourth processes, evoking and planning, are covered in Chapters 4 and 5.

AN OVERVIEW OF THE FOUR PROCESSES OF MI

The first process of MI is the act of engaging the client. The client is invited into a conversation that is warm and involves understanding how the client is feeling as a primary starting point. The counselor attempts to build rapport through posing inviting, nonthreatening, open-ended questions and uses reflective listening skills to demonstrate interest in understanding the client's story. Through the engaging process the counselor attempts to understand what the client is hoping to gain from the appointment. While the engaging process starts the session, the counselor aims to maintain that connection with the client throughout. Engaging the client isn't just about introducing oneself and finding out why the client made the appointment. It's about demonstrating from that very first moment that the client matters. This is demonstrated through being an attentive listener.

The second process involves helping the client to select a focus for the session. The client is asked what changes, if any, he or she is interested in making. Some clients arrive with a particular dietary or exercise change in mind that they'd like to try. Other clients have no idea what changes to make for a new diagnosis such as heart disease or diabetes. And others have little interest in making any changes. Considering all of the possibilities, it's important to allow clients to lead the focusing process. If a particular behavior change is not expressed by the client, the practitioner can provide various topics in the realm of nutrition and fitness and the client can select which topic is most appealing.

The third process, evoking, is centered on building motivation for change. The counselor asks open-ended questions that invite the client to explore reasons to change and how this change relates back to personal values. Evocation is part of the spirit of MI, and key in building motivation to change. Evoking questions are placed throughout a session with a primary purpose of promoting change talk, or phrases and sentences from clients that indicate interest in making a change.

Once the client seems ready for change, the conversation shifts to the fourth process, planning, which is discussing the "how to" of change. The client is invited to develop a plan of action and set specific, realistic goals to initiate a behavior change. In the spirit of MI and autonomy, the client leads this process. The practitioner asks the client how he or she might go about making the desired change and then is there to provide ideas, should the client need support.

The four processes are meant to provide structure and framing. They do not necessarily progress linearly, but do build on one another (see Figure 3.1). In ballroom dancing, a couple will cover different areas of the dance floor at different times during the dance. In MI, the practitioner and client work in much the same way. In addition, it is not necessary to work through each process in a single session, or even to progress in an exact order. For example, the counselor might begin by engaging the client and then invite her to focus on a specific topic. The counselor may ask the client evoking questions to elicit motivations for change. During the evoking process, the counselor may discover that the client is not particularly interested in making the behavior change originally selected and consequently they decide together to select a different focus.

In some appointments, the counselor and client may never discuss planning, especially if the client hasn't yet expressed readiness to change. In other sessions, the counselor and client may progress through evoking and planning and then decide to return to the focusing process when the client

			Planning
		Evoking	
	Focusing		
Engaging			
Engaging	**Focusing**	**Evoking**	**Planning**
• Give a warm, friendly greeting. • Make introductions. • Ask rapport-building questions. • Establish time available to meet. • Give an overview of what to expect. • Determine the reason for the visit.	• Invite the client to select a topic to discuss. • Present topic ideas to the client if the client is unsure. • Find out the reason behind topic selection.	• Identify and respond to ambivalence. • Evoke change talk. • Assess readiness to change. • Transition to planning process.	• Ask permission before giving information. • Offer information using elicit–provide–elicit. • Offer a concern. • Invite client to set goals • Assess barriers to change.

FIGURE 3.1. The four processes of MI. Based on Miller and Rollnick (2013).

selects a second behavior to change. Ultimately, the progression through the four processes depends on the client's motivation to change, which is fluid.

Ultimately, the progression through the four processes depends on the client's motivation to change, which is fluid.

The following brief MI session includes all four processes. In this example, the client is eager to make a specific behavior change. The counselor is able to guide the client through all four processes of the MI appointment, even with limited time.

Engaging

PRACTITIONER: Welcome, Annie. Glad you could make it. My name's Sue, and I'm a nutritionist. I was asked by your chiropractor to spend just 15–20 minutes with you today to discuss any nutrition topic that interests you. Before we get started, tell me a little about yourself.

CLIENT: Well, I'm 38 years old, live alone, and work at a local software company.

PRACTITIONER: So you work with computers. How do you like your job?

CLIENT: I've been there for about 8 years, and the job definitely has its perks. It's boring at times, but overall I enjoy the people I work with.

PRACTITIONER: It sounds like there are parts of it you enjoy, especially the people you work with. That's great!

PRACTITIONER: Before we get started, how did you feel about coming down to my office today?

CLIENT: Oh, not too bad. I wasn't sure what to expect; I've never met with a nutritionist before, but I saw your advertisement at my chiropractor's office and I thought I could really benefit from talking to someone.

PRACTITIONER: You're feeling like there might be some areas you could work on when it comes to your eating patterns and you're hoping I can help.

CLIENT: Yes. I mean, there's all this stuff on the Internet, but it's hard to figure out what is right. Plus, I thought meeting with someone would help me actually find the motivation.

PRACTITIONER: You're hoping that having someone to bounce ideas off of might help you make some changes to your diet.

CLIENT: Yes, it's nice to have some support.

PRACTITIONER: You're not completely sure what to expect, but you know you'd like some support as you attempt to make some changes that improve your health. I'd like to know a little more about the changes you're interested in making.

Focusing

PRACTITIONER: I have a chart here with seven different health topics we could discuss today and an empty circle in case there's something else that you'd like to discuss that's not on here. How do you feel about looking this over and deciding on a topic?

CLIENT: That would be fine. I was thinking on the way over here that it would be helpful to have someone to hold me accountable for this one change I've been meaning to make.

PRACTITIONER: Oh yeah? What's that?

CLIENT: I'd like to drink more water throughout the day.

Evoking

PRACTITIONER: You'd like to stay better hydrated. Tell me more about why you picked drinking more water as a change to work on.

CLIENT: Well, I drink a few sodas each week, coffee, and a little juice, but I was realizing the other day that I hardly ever drink water. I was reading a magazine article at the chiropractor's office the other day and it said that a lot of times people think they are hungry, but really they are just thirsty. I think I eat sometimes because I think I'm hungry, but I'm really just dehydrated.

PRACTITIONER: You're interested in drinking more water because you may be mistaking hunger for thirst.

CLIENT: Yes, exactly.

PRACTITIONER: What else motivates you to drink more water?

CLIENT: I've been feeling a cold coming on and I wonder if I drink more water if I would be able to fight off the cold better. Plus I've been feeling really run down lately; maybe I'm just dehydrated.

PRACTITIONER: You have a few different motivations for making this change. You mentioned that drinking more water might give you more energy, keep you from getting sick, and maybe even make you feel fuller. On a scale from 0 to 10, with 0 being uninterested and 10 being very interested, how interested are you in making this change?

CLIENT: I'd say I'm at about a 7 or an 8.

PRACTITIONER: A 7 or an 8 suggests you're pretty motivated to make this change. What led you to choose that number?

CLIENT: I'm really feeling like this change could benefit my health. However, I'm not quite sure how I'm going to go about actually adding more water to my day. Plus, I get bored with the taste of water, so it's hard to stay motivated to drink more.

PRACTITIONER: You have mixed feelings about making this change. On the one hand, you're concerned that adding more water might be a bit of a challenge, especially given that you aren't crazy about the taste and, on the other hand, you recognize how drinking more water might really help you stay well and have more energy.

CLIENT: Yes! It seems like a good change to make, but I know it won't be easy.

Planning

PRACTITIONER: You're willing to give it a try. What ideas do you have for increasing your water each day and making it taste good?

CLIENT: I have a water bottle, but I don't feel like grabbing it in the morning and filling it up. I think if I filled the bottle the night before and it already had cold water in it, I might be more inclined to take it with me when I go to work in the morning.

PRACTITIONER: So filling it up the night before might motivate you to be more consistent with your water bottle. What else?

CLIENT: I know if I just had it with me in the car and at work, I'd drink more water.

PRACTITIONER: You're pretty confident that if you had the water bottle with you in the morning, you would drink from it throughout the day. Would you like to hear another strategy that has worked for some of my clients?

CLIENT: Sure!

PRACTITIONER: Some have found that if they add flavoring to their water like lemons or a little juice, they are more likely to drink from their water bottles. You will be the best judge of whether something like this works for you. What are your thoughts?

CLIENT: Oh yes, I can see how that would help. I think the key is just remembering to get it all ready the night before. Maybe I can add fruit or juice to my water bottle and stick it in the fridge, and then I just need to remember to grab it in the morning.

PRACTITIONER: You've figured out a strategy that could work. What ideas do you have for reminders to grab your water out of the fridge in the morning?

CLIENT: Maybe if I just put a sign on the door out to the garage, I'll remember.

PRACTITIONER: Great idea! It sounds like you're excited to make this change. You've thought through the different ways this change might benefit your health and you have some strategies in mind for following through with your plan.

In this short script, the counselor leads the client across all areas of the dance floor, from the initial engaging interaction all the way to developing an action plan. However, it's the client who is coming up with the behavior change and plans for execution of the change. The counselor is simply inviting the client to consider motivators and barriers for making the change. This is a simplistic example, and in nutrition and fitness counseling, clients and conversations can be much more complicated. Remember that while the four processes provide a framework, because we're discussing human behavior, they cannot become formulaic. Ultimately, the processes and sequence of the appointment will largely depend on the client's needs.

The client's needs are assessed throughout the session. In many ways, the engage, focus, evoke, and plan of MI parallel the assessment, diagnosis, intervention, and monitor/evaluation of the Nutrition Care Process (NCP), which is highlighted in Figure 3.2. Similar to the NCP, in which assessment of the client guides the intervention, the engaging, focusing, and evoking steps lay the foundation and direction for the planning process. Traditionally, the practitioner has led the focusing process (nutrition diagnosis) of the appointment and provided strategies for making the behavior change. Alternatively, when using MI the client takes the lead on selecting a topic to focus on and is given the opportunity to come up with ways to make this change fit easily within his or her day-to-day schedule. The practitioner is there to help if the client runs out of ideas.

We will now go into more detail about implementing these four

NCP	MI Process	Examples
Assessment	Preappointment Engage Focus	• Practitioner reads medical chart. • Practitioner conducts an oral assessment. • Practitioner asks the client to complete an assessment questionnaire prior to the first visit. • Practitioner asks the client the reason for the visit. • Practitioner asks the client what he/she is hoping to get out of the session.
Diagnosis	Focus	• Practitioner asks client what changes, if any, he/she is interested in discussing further. • Practitioner shares possible topics to discuss based on assessment results. • Practitioner shares reason for consult, if unknown to the client.
Intervention	Evoking Planning	• Practitioner invites the client to voice motivations for behavior change. • Practitioner invites the client to determine a successful route toward change. • Practitioner guides the client to devise solutions for barriers to change. • Client determines specific goals for change.
Monitor/ evaluation	Planning Postappointment	• Practitioner invites the client to determine appropriate monitoring methods related to behavior change. • Practitioner and client discuss plans for follow-up. • Practitioner reviews any new lab values available.

FIGURE 3.2. MI and the NCP.

processes of MI, beginning with engaging and focusing in this chapter and evoking and planning in Chapters 4 and 5.

ENGAGING

It only takes about 3 seconds to make conclusions about a person we meet for the first time. In that short time we have a sense of whether the person can be trusted. What are qualities you look for in a potential friend, mentor, partner, or therapist in those first few seconds? A warm smile? Eye contact? A calming voice? Those initial qualities begin the engaging process.

The term *engage* means "to induce to participate" (*www.merriam-webster.com/dictionary/engage*). The goal of the engaging process is to establish a helpful connection. The first few minutes of an initial appointment or interaction serve as a foundation for all remaining interactions. Whether it's an initial phone call, or a warm, friendly greeting in the waiting room, those first exchanges set the tone for the rest of the session. As the counselor, you will send the client messages through words and body language, initiating the engaging process.

Clients can be engaged through both nonverbal and verbal communication. Nonverbal qualities to be aware of as a counselor include:

- *Body posture.* Maintain an open, relaxed posture, facing the client and leaning slightly forward to show you're paying attention.
- *Head nods.* Occasional head nods demonstrate agreement and encourage the client to continue to communicate. Excessive head nods can be distracting and can make you appear anxious or impatient.
- *Facial expressions.* It's important to appear natural, relaxed, and content. Be mindful of your emotional state; it's often exhibited through facial expressions. Some counselors find meditation and deep breathing exercises to be useful in centering oneself before a session.
- *Eye contact.* Comfort with eye contact varies between cultures. In Western cultures, maintaining eye contact demonstrates interest.
- *Voice.* Consider pitch, volume, tone, and speech clarity. Adopt a voice tone that is audible and clear, but not harsh or distracting.

What you verbally communicate to the client at the beginning of the appointment is also important in developing a counseling environment. The following are topics that could be included in the first few minutes of a session:

- Introduce yourself and inform the client of your role.
  "My name is Cheri and I'm a dietitian here at the clinic."

- Use open-ended questions to draw the client into a conversation.
  "Tell me a little about yourself."
  "What brings you in today?"

- Let the client know how much time you have for the session.
  "We have 30 minutes today to discuss your health habits."

- Give the client an overview of what to expect in the session.
  "I like to start out each session getting to know my client's eating and activity patterns. Then we can discuss how you feel about your current patterns and whether or not you're interested in making any changes. If you are interested in making a change, then we can discuss how you might set a specific goal for yourself."

- Ask permission to explore the client's thoughts and feelings surrounding food and fitness.
  "Would it be all right if we talked more about your thoughts and feelings surrounding food and activity today?"

Here's an example of an opening script that demonstrates the start of the engaging process. In this script an inpatient dietitian visits a patient who was recently diagnosed with congestive heart failure:

"Hi Jim, I'm Mike. I'm a dietitian here at the hospital. Your doctor asked that we meet to talk about your new dietary needs to protect your heart. I have about 15 minutes today to begin talking about that. If our time today isn't enough, I can return tomorrow, or we can schedule an appointment for you to see our clinic dietitian the next time you visit your doctor. Would it be all right with you if we talked for a little bit about food and health? . . . Tell me a little about yourself and what you're hoping to get out of our time together." [The practitioner then spends 2–3 minutes listening, finding out how the client is feeling, and uses core MI skills to convey an understanding of this.]

In just a few sentences, this dietitian has introduced himself, explained his role, and the time allotted. He has asked the client's permission to discuss nutrition and has engaged him with a simple open-ended question. Working at the beginning of the appointment to build rapport with the client is time well spent. The engaging process is like laying a foundation on which a house can be built. If great care is taken to make a strong, solid, smooth foundation, then there will be fewer problems with the house. In a well-laid MI foundation, there is a sense of trust between client and counselor. A weak foundation, laid in haste, could result in the client feeling judged or pressured to change, and shutting down without gaining anything from his time with you.

6

LISTENING

ask ourselves which person in our lives means the ~ often find that it is those who, instead of giving much ~utions, or cures, have chosen rather to share our pain and ~n our wounds with a gentle and tender hand.

—HENRI NOUWEN

The key to building a strong foundation is to be a good listener. Ultimately, engaging the client is not following a certain script or asking the client questions, but listening, *really listening.* Listen with your eyes, your body, and your words. Listen with delight and curiosity (see Figure 3.3). Give the client your complete, undivided attention. An experienced counselor is able to maintain not only a physical presence, but an emotional presence. This is only possible when the counselor is able to put aside the mental to-do list and focus on the client.

A client feels heard when the counselor not only looks attentive, but also provides verbal responses, or reflections, of what the client is saying. We provide a more in-depth discussion of reflections in Chapter 8. At times, simple encouragers such as "Mmmm-hmmm," or "I see," or "Tell me more" are all that are needed to engage the client. At other times, listening involves maintaining complete eye contact and presence, but also silence, allowing the client to express all that is on his mind. While extended silence may seem awkward, some clients may require more processing time. Experienced counselors are comfortable with silence. Moments when no one is talking are moments in which the client has more time to process or to respond. We have two ears, two eyes, and one mouth, and when we use them in that same ratio (80% listening, 20% talking), clients feel heard and respected.

> *We have two ears, two eyes, and one mouth, and when we use them in that same ratio (80% listening, 20% talking), clients feel heard and respected.*

There are three benefits to being a good listener. First, listening engages the client and builds trust, loyalty, and commitment in the relationship. Through paraphrasing or reflecting what the client says in a genuine fashion, you will display empathy for the client's situation. When a client feels heard, he is likely to share more personal information. By being a good listener, you can show you care. Second, clients often experience emotional healing or reduced anxiety about a behavior change just through talking about their concerns. When people feel heard, they want to talk more; they feel understood, respected, and accepted. There is something therapeutic about talking. You may, in fact, need to say very little at times for the client to reach his own resolutions. Third, through being a good listener, you will be able to better assess the situation and consequently provide better behavior change counseling.

Listen with:
- Presence
- Undivided attention
- Eyes, ears, and heart
- Acceptance
- Curiosity
- Delight
- Silence
- Words

FIGURE 3.3. Listening. Adapted with permission from MI training materials used by Steven M. Berg-Smith.

Listening is the greatest gift a counselor can give to a client. As Carl Rogers once said, "I don't know what it is about listening. I just know when I'm heard, it feels damned good."

REENGAGING

Even if you succeed in engaging a client at the beginning of a session, it's possible to lose engagement later in the appointment. You may start to lose engagement if the client hears something that rubs him the wrong way or is not of interest. You may notice a shift in the client's posture, eye contact, mood, or he will become quiet or agitated. When this happens, you can re-engage him by simply checking in. The following practitioner statements can be used to draw the client back in:

"I get the feeling that I've said something that's made you uncomfortable. What's going on for you right now?"
"I can sense that you don't like that suggestion I just made."
"Let me check in with you. What are your thoughts and feelings about what I just said?"
"I feel as though I might have lost you. Perhaps we need to back up or switch gears. What are your thoughts?"

It may be tempting to ignore the fact that you and your client are no longer on the same page. You could continue on in the conversation pretending as if the connection was not lost, but if you do that, there is a chance the client may begin to tune out, or stop caring about the behavior change at hand.

Overall, engaging a client is about building a connection. This is accomplished through asking the client specific questions about his or her initial hopes and expectations for a session and then listening with your whole body, while demonstrating components of the spirit of MI such as empathy, compassion, and partnership.

FOCUSING

Once the client is engaged, she can be guided to select a topic or behavior to focus on. Sometimes right away the client voices a behavior to change. Other times the client knows she wants help changing her eating or activity patterns, but doesn't know where to start. When this is the case, you can provide her with a list of possibilities, known as agenda mapping (Miller & Rollnick, 2013). You and the client discuss possible topics and decide together which direction might be best. Typically, within this brief focusing conversation, you ask the client for topic ideas and also present a menu of options that you believe might apply to the client's situation. Once you have a map of various behavior change destinations, you can discuss an agenda. Which topics might be useful to address first? Second? Eventually?

When providing topic ideas, it's important to offer the right number of options. Too many choices, and the client could become overwhelmed. Too few, and she could feel forced into a behavior change that she is not interested in.

It can be helpful to use a visual aide as you discuss possible topics. Stott and colleagues used this method in their diabetes education (Stott, Rollnick, Rees, & Pill, 1995). Circle charts, also known as bubble sheets, were used to introduce possible topics (see Handout 3.1). A circle chart is simply a piece of paper with several circles, each with a different topic. Circle charts are preferred over lists because topics are not provided in any order, and therefore no one topic is seen as more important or necessary than another.

Clients like to have options. A well-made circle chart includes at least one blank circle for the client to write in a topic that is not present. In addition, it is important to give clients an out. While showing the client the circle chart, ask him, "Which, if any, of these topics interest you?" By using the words "if any," you give the client freedom to express a lack of interest in making a change, or to present a new topic.

You can introduce circle charts with an informal question—for example, "Would you like to see a list of topics that I have discussed with some of my other clients? Which, if any, of these topics interest you?"

You may find it useful to have a variety of circle charts for various disease states or conditions. A client who is being seen by a child feeding expert may select a topic from a circle chart that is designed for parents or parents-to-be, with circles on such topics as:

Handout 3.1

CIRCLE CHART FOR NUTRITION AND FITNESS COUNSELING

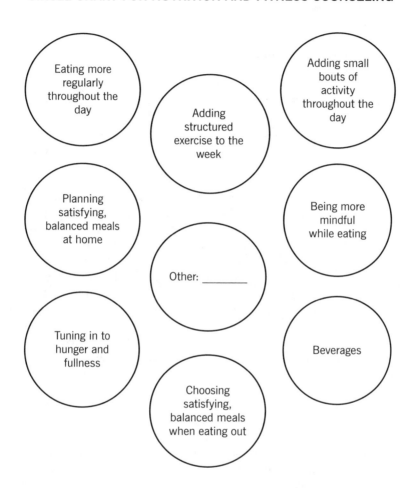

1. Picky eaters
2. Overeating
3. Undereating
4. Planning meals and snacks
5. Managing child behavior at the table
6. Breastfeeding/weaning
7. Baby's first foods

Once the client selects a topic, or suggests an alternative topic, reflect the choice. Follow up the reflection with an open-ended question to find out more about why the client has selected that particular behavior—for example, "You're concerned your daughter isn't eating enough and you'd like to discuss strategies for increasing her intake. Tell me more about your choice."

Nutrition and fitness professionals are notorious for trying to cover too many topics in one session. Making a single behavior change can be quite a task. It's best to tackle one topic at a time and work through motivations and barriers for that single topic. It's better if the client is confident in making one change than less confident in making several changes at once. Each behavior change success increases client confidence in reaching future health goals. You can pull out the circle chart again in future sessions as the client masters a behavior change and feels ready to attempt new changes.

> *It's better if the client is confident in making one change than less confident in making several changes at once.*

FOCUSING STYLES

When assessing the client, it may become clear which behavior change would benefit the client most, which would align with the nutrition diagnosis step of the NCP. If the practitioner chooses the focus of the session, then it is considered a counselor-directed session.

However, when incorporating motivational interviewing into the session, the client might be asked to choose the nutritional problem he or she would like to work on, thereby making the nutritional diagnosis and intervention client driven. With permission, the practitioner would share her opinion about which change or changes will most likely result in the outcomes the client desires. Sometimes the client selects a behavior change that lines up with the nutrition-related problem that the practitioner feels is most important. However, this is not always the case.

Let's say that following the assessment, the nutrition practitioner is convinced that the most important nutritional problem for a client with hypertension is his low intake of potassium-rich foods (as evidenced by low serum potassium and the dietary recall). After asking permission, she tells the client that increasing intake of potassium-rich fruits and vegetables is the most effective way to address his blood pressure and provides an additional list of other possible behaviors on which to focus for lowering blood pressure, such as physical activity and reducing dietary sodium. What if the client has no interest in adding potassium-rich foods, but instead is interested in increasing physical activity? What should the practitioner do? Explain the importance of the practitioner-selected nutritional diagnosis (inadequate intake of potassium), or head in the direction selected by the client? Hang on to that question for a minute while you consider the following.

There are three styles in determining the focus and therefore the primary nutritional diagnosis addressed in the session: directing, following, and guiding. If the practitioner uses a directing style, then the practitioner decides on the focus of the session and doesn't ask for the client's input. Directing would sound like this:

> "As I mentioned, your blood potassium levels are low, which is likely a result of the diuretic you're taking. It's important to get your potassium levels back up. In addition, eating potassium-rich fruits and vegetables may help lower your blood pressure. Let's talk about that today."

If the practitioner uses a following style, then the practitioner gives the client full rein in selecting the focus, as in the following example:

> PRACTITIONER: Now that I've explained the different changes that clients with high blood pressure often make, which one, if any, sounds most appealing to you right now?
>
> CLIENT: I've been wanting to start exercising again, so I think I'd like to start with that one.
>
> PRACTITIONER: Great. What ideas do you have?

If the practitioner uses a guiding style, then both parties are involved in discussing and deciding upon the focus. Guiding would sound like this:

> PRACTITIONER: Now that I've explained the different changes that clients with high blood pressure often make, which one sounds most appealing to you right now?
>
> CLIENT: I've been wanting to start exercising again, so I think I'd like to start with that one.
>
> PRACTITIONER: You'd like to start looking at ways to be more active. We can certainly explore that some more. May I share my thoughts

about how your recent lab tests might help us choose the most effective things to do?

CLIENT: Sure.

PRACTITIONER: The lab tests here are telling me your blood potassium levels are low. Adding high-potassium foods into your diet would bring these values up and help your blood pressure. What is your response to this?

CLIENT: Yes, that concerns me too. It would be good to talk about that also. I know bananas are high in potassium, but I'm sure there are other foods you could tell me about.

PRACTITIONER: Yes, I have a list here we can look at if you're interested. Perhaps we could start today's session by talking about your plans for exercise and then before you leave we can revisit potassium. How does that sound?

Guiding is a collaborative approach that acknowledges that the client's agenda and the practitioner's expertise are both important. This method best aligns with MI while still addressing the nutrition diagnosis that becomes apparent in the nutrition assessment. By giving the client the option to select the focus of the session, you maintain a spirit of autonomy and choice, which may increase the client's reception to discussing other topics in the future. In addition, if the client starts by making a change he is confident he can make, this confidence may help him succeed when he attempts other health-related behavior changes.

REFOCUSING

On occasion, the conversation may begin drifting away from the topic of the behavior change. When this happens, you may need to reengage the client and help to refocus the conversation. In the following script, notice how the practitioner brings the client back by bringing up the original focus and then asking an open-ended question. There's more on open-ended questions in Chapter 6.

PRACTITIONER: You picked "meal planning" on the circle chart as a topic you'd like to address in this appointment. Tell me more about why you selected that topic.

CLIENT: I've been eating out a lot. I went to this one restaurant the other day and you wouldn't believe the portions they served! I wanted to split a meal with my wife, but she wanted to order oysters. I don't like oysters. The last time I ate oysters was during this cruise we took 10 years ago and I got really sick. I was sick for 7 of the 10 days we were on the boat. My poor wife had to go do all of the activities without me while I lay in bed. Talk about cabin fever! Those rooms are so small, and when you're not feeling well . . . it was the pits.

PRACTITIONER: That must have put a real damper on your vacation. You mentioned some unfortunate eating out experiences. Help me understand how your recent eating out experiences inspired you to do more meal planning.

In this example, the practitioner acknowledges the client's story and gently draws him back into the focus of the appointment.

While the practitioner and client never really leave the engaging process, they do move on into other processes. With a specific behavior change in mind the conversation can transition gracefully into evoking and planning to discuss the motivators and "how to's" of change.

CHAPTER 4

Evoking

What people really need is a good listening to.
—MARY LOU CASEY

The third process of MI is evoking. Here, the practitioner uses open-ended questions to invite the client to consider personal interest and motivations for a behavior change.

While making a healthy behavior change may seem like the right thing to do, there are many cogent and convincing reasons *not* to change. Therefore, clients are often conflicted about adopting new behaviors. In the evoking process, the practitioner guides the client to examine this ambivalence toward change. The practitioner uses evocative questions to bring to light the client's mixed feelings about change.

Evocative questions are asked in a nonjudgmental fashion, supporting that it is ultimately the client's decision whether to change. The goal of the evoking process is to inspire motivation. Telling a client why he should change is often ineffective in promoting long-lasting behavior change. Instead, an MI practitioner invites a client to voice his personal motivations for change. While evoking may occur throughout the counseling sessions, evoking change talk, which we defined in Chapter 1 as comments made by the client that support change, is especially useful before the "how to change" or planning is discussed.

Telling a client why he should change is often ineffective in promoting long-lasting behavior change.

Counseling strategies we review in this chapter include identifying and responding to ambivalence, evoking language from the client about change, assessing readiness to change, and transitioning the client to the fourth process, planning.

MOVING THROUGH AMBIVALENCE

It's normal to have mixed feelings about change. When a client is ambivalent or contemplative about a certain behavior, help him take a look at this behavior from different angles. While helping the client explore ambivalence, it is important to do so without judgment or bias. If a client feels pressured into working on a particular behavior change, you may find his motivation fizzles. Maintain an aura of curiosity and exploration. The client will then feel comfortable being honest with his feelings and opinions surrounding the issue at hand.

Identifying Ambivalence

How can you tell if your client is ambivalent? You can detect his ambivalence in his verbal and nonverbal communication. Pay close attention to the client's spoken words, his facial expressions, and his body language to assess ambivalence.

When you ask a client to discuss his feelings about making a behavior change, his responses typically fall into one of two categories: change talk or sustain talk. Change talk is when the client expresses a desire to change, comments on his ability to change, mentions a reason and need for change, or shares a commitment to change. In addition, the client may already be actively taking steps to change. A simple acronym can help you recall what change talk sounds like: DARN CAT, which stands for Desire, Ability, Reason, Need, Commitment, Activation, and Taking steps (Rollnick , Miller, & Butler, 2008; see Figure 4.1).

The "DARN" part of the acronym represents *preparatory* change talk, whereas the "CAT" part represents *mobilizing* change talk. At first, a client

---

DARN CAT

Desire to change: "I really want to stop binging."

Abilities to change: "I can do this."

Reasons to change: "If I stop binging, I won't feel as bloated."

Needs for change: "I need to stop binging—it makes me feel bloated in the morning."

Commitment to change: "I am going to start eating more throughout the day so I don't feel like binging at night."

Activation: "I bought some snack foods that I feel safe with."

Taking Steps: "I didn't binge the other day, even though we had Halloween candy in the house."

FIGURE 4.1. Change talk.

may only express preparatory change talk, but as he becomes more interested in making a behavior change, you may begin to hear more mobilizing change talk (see Figure 4.2).

A second category is sustain talk, which is a client's statement that favors the status quo over movement toward change. Here are examples of client statements that are considered sustain talk:

> "I just can't eat breakfast, because I don't feel hungry in the morning."
> "I *need* my energy drink in the morning or else I just feel "off" the rest of the day."
> "I can't afford a gym membership, and it's not safe in my neighborhood to walk."
> "I know how many carbohydrates are in rice, but I can't give it up. It's my main dish."

You can identify ambivalence when change talk and sustain talk are both present in client comments. For example, a client might say, "I know I need to change the way I eat. I can't live like this anymore. I just can't get on track, though. I am good all day long and then one thing goes wrong and I blow it. I don't know what goes wrong; I just can't control myself. What can I say, I like food. I just do." In this client response, both sustain talk and

Preparatory change talk		Mobilizing change talk	
Client statement	Type (DARN CAT)	Client statement	Type (DARN CAT)
"I don't want to end up like my uncle who had a heart attack."	Desire	"I'm going to start training with my girlfriend for a 10K run."	Commitment
"I've cut down on soda before, so I know I can do it again."	Ability	"I'm willing to cut back my eating out habit to 3 days a week."	Activation
"I hate the fact that the gym makes money off of me because I never go."	Reason	"I bought a new swimsuit that would be perfect for doing some laps."	Taking steps
"I really need to cut back on the amount of caffeine I drink. I think it's affecting my sleep at night."	Need		

FIGURE 4.2. Examples of preparatory and mobilizing change talk.

change talk are present. Comments such as "I can't live like this anymore" sound like change talk, whereas "I just can't control myself" and "What can I say, I like food" exemplify sustain talk. Some clients may be aware of and surprisingly honest about their ambivalence; others may be less aware.

Obvious Ambivalence

At times, clients are quite honest and up-front regarding their mixed feelings. For example, a client may state, "I know I'm supposed to work out all the time, but it's too hard to stick with it, so I don't even know why I bother."

No Signs of Ambivalence

Often clients are unaware of the challenges involved with a behavior change, and come across overly confident. For example, a client may state, "I'm tired of feeling so tired all the time. So I'm really hoping you can help me change my diet. I'm willing to do whatever it takes. Just give me a plan and I'll do it!" Overly ambitious clients can be ambivalent on the inside, but eager to please their practitioners. Therefore, even with an eager client, it can be useful to invite her to explore motivations for change.

Mixed Messages

Clients may express verbally that they are ready to make a behavior change, but their non-verbal cues suggest otherwise. For example, a client might say, "Sure, I guess I could try that." But at the same she is making inconsistent eye contact, shrugging, blowing out long sighs, or making negative facial expressions. These nonverbal cues may be signs that the client is not ready to change.

Below is a series of brief clinical dialogues demonstrating the different forms of ambivalence.

Obvious Ambivalence

CLIENT 1: I know I'm supposed to work out all the time, but it's too hard to stick with it, so I don't even know why I bother.

PRACTITIONER: You've noticed that it's challenging to maintain a regular exercise routine with your busy schedule, and you're aware that exercising has many benefits. You'd like to experience those benefits again.

CLIENT 1: Yes. I know that when I was younger and I was running regularly, I felt like a million bucks. I had more energy and I just felt better about myself in general.

PRACTITIONER: You'd like to get back to that place.

No Signs of Ambivalence

CLIENT 2: I'm tired of feeling so tired all the time. So I'm really hoping you can help me change my diet. I'm willing to do whatever it takes. Just give me a plan and I'll do it!

PRACTITIONER: You're motivated to make a change that improves your energy. What else is important to you about making this change?

CLIENT 2: I just don't think I'm getting the nutrition I need since I eat out all the time. I want to be healthier.

PRACTITIONER: Your health is important to you. How would your life be different if you did decide to change up your diet a bit?

CLIENT 2: I'd probably have to start cooking more. I'm a pretty decent cook, I've just gotten lazy lately and it has been easier to eat out. But the foods I'm eating at restaurants are not the healthiest and I always leave restaurants feeling sluggish and bloated.

PRACTITIONER: While eating out is easier, you see yourself cooking more because you feel better when you eat meals at home.

Mixed Messages

PRACTITIONER: What ideas do you have for quick easy snacks to eat right after your practices?

CLIENT 3: I have no idea. What are athletes supposed to eat after workouts?

PRACTITIONER: Some of my clients have found it easiest to keep nonperishable foods in their lockers like granola bars or trail mix. That way they can get started on refueling their muscles right after practice. What are your thoughts on that idea?

CLIENT 3: Sure, I guess I could try that.

PRACTITIONER: It sounds like you're somewhat interested, but I also get the feeling that you have some hesitations.

CLIENT 3: Yeah, it could work, but I'm sure the guys will give me a hard time about it in the locker room.

PRACTITIONER: It sounds like loading up your locker with food isn't exactly "cool."

CLIENT 3: No. And while they're making fun of me, they'll be asking me for some too.

PRACTITIONER: Yes, and I bet you don't want to be giving away all of your food. Those are some legitimate concerns. You'd like to increase your performance and you recognize that eating after practice might help. You also have some barriers to making it happen. What ideas do you have?

CLIENT 3: I could keep food in my car.

PRACTITIONER: Great idea. By keeping food in your car, maybe you wouldn't have to worry about your teammates.

Responding to Ambivalence

In the examples above, the practitioner responded to change talk and sustain talk by repeating back pieces of what the client was saying. Reflective listening is an excellent way to cue clients into their ambivalence. Following are some specific strategies for responding to ambivalence. More examples of reflective listening are provided in Chapter 8.

Reflecting Both Sides

When you hear or see ambivalence, it's useful to reflect both sides of it. For example, the practitioner responded to Client 1 above with, "You've noticed that it's challenging to maintain a regular exercise routine with your busy schedule, and you're aware that exercising has many benefits. You'd like to experience those benefits again." In this reflection, the practitioner mentions both the sustain talk and the change talk; therefore, the client hears that she has mixed feelings about the behavior.

Emphasizing Change Talk

While it's appropriate at times to reflect both the sustain talk and change talk to help the client see she has mixed feelings about change, it's best to focus most of your reflective listening statements on the change talk. If the client expresses change talk, or even hints at change talk, highlight that piece when reflecting.

In the Client 1 example above, the practitioner ends the reflection on a positive note, taking a guess that the client is interested in the benefits of exercise. By ending with the change talk, the client is focused on that piece and may well continue to speak of the benefits experienced when she was younger. Instead of dwelling on having a hard time fitting exercise into her busy schedule, she is moving forward by focusing on feeling better when she is active.

Here's another example of a client statement followed by a practitioner response that highlights the change talk:

CLIENT: Giving up my energy drinks is going to be hard. I'll probably be dragging for a few days. But I quit smoking a few years ago and nothing can be as hard as that was.

PRACTITIONER: You recognize that while it may be hard at first, you know you have what it takes to make this change.

This is another example of how highlighting the client's change talk builds motivation and affirms that he has what it takes to make a behavior change.

Evoking Change Talk

In the evoking process the practitioner asks strategic open-ended questions to elicit change talk from the client and then highlights the change talk using reflective listening techniques. In asking these evocative open-ended questions, the practitioner invites the client to consider his personal motivation for change and how making this change might improve his life. The following open-ended questions are useful in evoking change talk:

"What was it like to receive that diagnosis?"
"What are the best and worst parts?"
"What is important to you about this change? What does it mean to you?"
"What would have to be different for the importance to be higher?"
"How would your life be different after this change?"
"How might this particular change get you what you want?"
"What concerns do you have about what you are doing now? What bothers you most about it?"
"What *don't* you like about [negative behavior]?"
"Who would be able to support you in this change? Who would like this change?"
"How is what you're doing right now not working for you?"
"How would your life be different if you did decide to make changes?"
"How would changing make your life better?"

While the majority of questions asked in the evoking process are to elicit change talk, now and then the practitioner may ask a question with the intention of eliciting sustain talk. Examples of evocative questions that elicit sustain talk include:

"What might make it hard for you to make this change?"
"What do you like about your current way of doing things?"

These types of questions may be used now and then to invite the client to consider current barriers to making a behavior change. However, the goal of an MI session is to elicit as much change talk as possible. Therefore, use questions that elicit sustain talk sparingly.

PUTTING THE PIECES TOGETHER:
EVOKING AND REFLECTING CHANGE TALK

The following dialogue includes three of the four processes of MI. The appointment begins with engaging, followed by focusing. Once the client has selected a specific behavior he is interested in changing, the practitioner attempts to build motivation by evoking and reflecting change talk. Throughout this dialogue the change talk is **bolded** and the sustain talk is underlined.

Engaging

PRACTITIONER: What brings you in today? [open-ended question]

CLIENT: I'm just here because my doctor told me he wanted me to try changing my diet before he puts me on those drugs to lower my cholesterol. (*Voice tone sounds unenthusiastic.*)

PRACTITIONER: OK, so you're here because your doctor referred you for help lowering your cholesterol through diet and exercise. [reflection] How do you feel about being here? [open-ended question]

CLIENT: I don't know. **He doesn't know that I already tried making changes a year ago when I was with my last doctor** and it was impossible.

PRACTITIONER: You tried making changes on your own; you obviously care about your health. [affirmation] Tell me more about that. [open-ended question]

CLIENT: **Yeah, it's not like I want a heart attack or anything.** I just don't have time to eat all perfect, so I wish he'd just give me those drugs already.

PRACTITIONER: You're aware of the risks of high cholesterol and having a heart attack is one risk that concerns you. [reflection]

CLIENT: **Yeah, I would like to stick around a little longer. I'm good at popping pills.** It's the whole cooking thing that gets me. Plus, I like food, and I like to eat and you're just going to tell me to stop eating, or something.

PRACTITIONER: You're someone who is consistent when it comes to taking medication, so you feel that might be your most viable option at this point. You're concerned that making changes to lower your cholesterol would involve having to eliminate foods you like. You seem to care about your health and want to improve your cholesterol. I appreciate your honesty in sharing some reservations you had about seeing me today. Some of my clients have found that by making a few small changes, they've been able to lower their cholesterol without having to revamp their entire diets. Even making a few small changes can be hard, though. Ultimately, it's your choice what you'd like to do. [summary]

Focusing

PRACTITIONER: We have about 30 minutes to spend together today and I'm wondering how I can best help you. [open-ended question]

CLIENT: <u>You can help me by telling my doctor just to give me those pills!</u>

PRACTITIONER: I'd be happy to talk to your doctor about that. How else can I help? [open-ended question]

CLIENT: I don't know. I eat out a lot, and I can't really cook all that great, so maybe just **tell me what foods I can order, or something**.

PRACTITIONER: What's most feasible for you right now is to maybe make a few changes in the foods you order when you eat out. [reflection] You've come up with a change that feels doable to you. [affirmation] Tell me more about the foods you like to order at a restaurant. What are your favorites? [open-ended question]

CLIENT: I like a good burger and French fries. I also get burritos from the Mexican restaurant near my work. Now and then I hit up a sandwich shop, and I get pizza and beer with the guys on Friday nights. Oh, and I just started going to this new BBQ place a few blocks from my apartment where the ribs are something else! I just start salivating when I think about them.

PRACTITIONER: You have many restaurant favorites. [reflection] Before we start talking about finding a few small changes in what you order to lower your cholesterol, can we talk for a moment about your health concerns? [asking permission]

CLIENT: Yeah, that's fine.

Evoking

PRACTITIONER: You mentioned earlier that you don't want to have a heart attack. [summary] What else motivates you to make choices that support your health right now? [open-ended question to evoke more change talk]

CLIENT: I have this new girlfriend who's pretty special. We really have a good time together. And things are just getting good, so **I don't want to die on her.**

PRACTITIONER: There's someone special in your life who might miss you. [reflection of change talk]

CLIENT: Yeah, she wanted to come today, but had to be somewhere else. When I told her about this cholesterol stuff, she was like, "You're stubborn as hell; I don't know how that dietitian is going to get you to do anything with your diet." She knows me pretty well, doesn't she?

PRACTITIONER: It's nice when the people we care about "get" us. [affirmation] I'm not really interested in talking you into doing anything you don't want to do. It's your health and your body, and you get to decide how you want to treat it. I'm just here if you want help. [demonstration of autonomy]

CLIENT: **Yeah, it can't hurt to make a few changes,** <u>as long as I still get to eat my ribs.</u>

PRACTITIONER: Yes, let's be sure to keep those as part of your diet. They sound pretty important to you. [reflection]

CLIENT: They'd be important to you too if you had tried them.

PRACTITIONER: I'll have to be sure and do that. What else motivates you to want to treat your body right? [open-ended question to evoke change talk]

CLIENT: I've seen some close friends go through the wringer lately in terms of their health. **I don't want the last few decades to be a miserable existence. I want to get out and do things when I retire.**

PRACTITIONER: You'd like to stay active in your older years, and you believe taking care of yourself now might pay off later. [reflection of change talk]

CLIENT: **Yes, plus these doctors' visits cost a fortune and that's one fortune I won't have as I get older.**

PRACTITIONER: Cost of medical bills if your health declines also motivates you to stay healthy. [reflection of change talk]

CLIENT: Yeah, I have a hard enough time as it is making my bills each month; **I don't need medical debt.**

PRACTITIONER: Thank you for explaining what motivates you to change. [affirmation] You mentioned that being healthy and active for your girlfriend are important, as well as cost. [summary] What else? [open-ended question to evoke change talk]

CLIENT: Can't think of anything. I lead a pretty simple life.

PRACTITIONER: At this point, how important is it to you to make some small changes in your ordering habits when you eat out? [open-ended question to assess readiness to change]

CLIENT: **I'd say it's pretty important.** As long as I can treat myself to an occasional rib dinner, **then it shouldn't be too bad.**

At the beginning of this dialogue, the client expresses significant sustain talk and some change talk. The practitioner reflects the client's ambivalence while also emphasizing his change talk. As a result, the client expresses more change talk. In addition, the practitioner strategically evokes more change talk by asking questions such as "What motivates you to take care of your health?" The practitioner does not push the client into making a change he isn't interested in making. Instead, she promotes client choice in selecting a behavior change that feels doable.

PREPARING FOR PLANNING

In the previous dialogue, the practitioner begins to hear significant change talk toward the end of the conversation and then asks how important the change is to the client. Assessing readiness is an important step before diving into the planning process. If the client values the new behavior, then he is more likely to be ready to attempt the change.

If the client values the new behavior, then he is more likely to be ready to attempt the change.

Another way to assess the client's readiness to change is to use a scaling question. Scaling questions invite clients to consider their level of interest or readiness to change on a scale from 0 to 10, with 10 meaning fully ready or interested and 0 meaning not at all ready or interested.

Here are some examples of scaling questions you can use to assess a client's readiness to change:

"On a scale from 0 to 10, with 0 being 'not at all' and 10 being 'very,'
   'how important is this change to you?'
   'how confident are you that you can make this change?'
   'how interested are you in making this change at this time?'
   'how ready are you to make this change?' "

In general, scaling questions that ask about interest or importance occur more at the beginning of the appointment when discussing motivations for change, while a scaling question regarding confidence in making the change is typically asked more toward the end of the session after the planning has been discussed.

Once a scaling question is asked, follow-up questions are useful in exploring reasons behind the answer. It is important to find out why the client selected a particular number to represent her readiness to change before moving forward.

The following script demonstrates how to use a scaling question to assess readiness to change.

> PRACTITIONER: At this point you've shared some specific reasons why you would like to bring your lunch to work more often, including the fact that it will save you money and result in a lower-sodium meal. And you've also expressed that it may be a bit challenging at first to get the hang of putting that lunch together in the morning. [summary] I'm curious at this point, how interested are you on a scale from 0 to 10 to begin bringing your lunch to work a few times a week? 10 would mean that you are eager and ready to make this change and 0 would mean that you're really quite hesitant. [scaling question]
>
> CLIENT: I'm at about a 7 or an 8.
>
> PRACTITIONER: OK, a 7 or 8. So you're somewhat ready to make this change. [reflection] Tell me a little bit about your answer. Why not a 6? Or why not higher, like a 9? [open-ended probing question]
>
> CLIENT: Well, I'm fairly confident that I want to make this change. I came up with the idea in the first place, so there's a big part of me that wants to give it a try. But I guess I'm not a 9 or a 10 because we haven't quite talked through how exactly it's going to go or what types of foods I will need to bring with me. So I'm a little nervous about the unknown at this point. Plus, I know I'm going to want to eat out with my coworkers whenever I'm invited to. So I can see how that's going to be a little tricky.
>
> PRACTITIONER: OK, so you're a little concerned about how you'll handle the social aspect of the change and how you'll make time to prepare your lunch in the morning, and this is still a change you'd like to test out because you believe it will improve your health. [reflection]

Once it is apparent that the client is ready to change, the discussion can begin to shift toward action planning. Summaries can be useful when transitioning clients to the "how-to" or "information giving" part of the counseling session. In a summary at the end of the building motivation process, revisit the main points of what the client has shared. Include:

- The original reason the appointment was made.
- Interesting information that was uncovered that seems pertinent.
- A few key reasons the client would like to change.
- Any major concerns the client has about change.
- The client's general readiness to change.

This kind of summary helps the client organize his thoughts. It also provides another opportunity for you to check in with her to make sure she is feeling heard and understood. A summary will also help transition to the planning process of the appointment. More information about summaries can be found in Chapter 9.

After a brief summary, invite the client to consider how she might make the change. You may ask, "How do you think you'll go about making this change?" This question provides the client an opportunity to think through the "how to" on her own first, and is known in the MI field as "the key question." It signifies transition from the evoking process to the planning process. Through asking this specific open-ended question you invite the client to have the first stab at problem solving, giving the client autonomy. In the following dialogue, the practitioner provides a summary followed by an open-ended question to transition to the planning process.

PRACTITIONER: I'd like to take a minute to recap what we've talked about so far, if it's OK with you.

CLIENT: Sure.

PRACTITIONER: You made this appointment today because you'd like to lose weight. We talked about different diets you've been on and how those haven't worked, and they've often left you feeling worse about yourself in the end. You're interested in making some changes that are more personalized for your life. For starters, you'd like to eat out less often. You believe it will save you money and you won't feel as full after meals. You're worried that it will take more time on the weekends to shop and plan for meals. You're also excited about the opportunity to eat more fruits and vegetables and foods that make your body feel good. What did I miss? [transitional summary]

CLIENT: Nothing. That sounds about right.

PRACTITIONER: With this change of eating out less often, what ideas do you have for how this could work for you? [open-ended question]

What Do I Do When My Patient Cries?

Evoking often results in an emotional response, especially when the topic is body image or disordered eating. Therefore, before working with clients, create an environment where crying is viewed as a normal emotional response and fully accepted. Keep those tissues handy! When a client tears up, it's important to acknowledge that he or she is expressing emotion, and to find out where those feelings emerge from. One common response is, "I'm noticing some emotion as we discuss your frustrations with losing and gaining weight. Tell me about that." When you acknowledge the emotion in a neutral manner, the client receives the message that it is acceptable to express what he or she is feeling, and is invited to consider how feelings influence her behavior.

Often when a client is emotional, there is more beneath the surface to explore and uncover. On occasion, topics may arise that are beyond the capabilities of the nutrition or fitness practitioner, warranting a referral to a psychotherapist (see Appendix 1). When you take the time to really understand all the elements of what the client is experiencing, both verbal and nonverbal cues, these internal conflicts can float to the surface; and if the client is ready to explore these emotions, great healing can take place.

Pitfalls of Jumping the Gun

A common mistake of nutrition and fitness practitioners is to jump to the planning process too quickly. Practitioners are often eager to start teaching the client new skills or brainstorming strategies for making the change easy. Skipping the evoking process is especially tempting when there is little time for the session, or when the practitioner doesn't expect to see the client for future appointments. However, the cost of jumping to the planning process too quickly is that the client leaves the practitioner's office with a plan but with low motivation to follow through. The client is then less likely to make any changes, which can result in discouragement about behavior changes altogether.

The amount of time spent in the evoking and planning processes depends on clients' readiness to change, and varies greatly between clients. Some clients express excitement about a particular behavior change. With these types of clients, you may only need to spend a few minutes in the evoking process. Often, however, clients express overconfidence in their abilities to change. Therefore, it is still important to briefly explore with even the most seemingly motivated clients any hesitations, concerns, or potential barriers to change.

For other clients, a great deal of time may be spent eliciting change talk. Clients less eager to change may need to spend several appointments in the evoking process. For a client who is referred to a dietitian and states,

"I'm only here because my doctor made me come," it may be helpful to spend more time exploring the client's concerns about his health.

The engaging, focusing, and evoking processes are important prepping steps for the planning process. Let's say you were going to paint a room in your house. What's the first step? Preparing the walls. Holes in the wall may need to be filled, texturing may need to be done, and blue tape applied around windows, walls and ceilings. The preparation step of painting is the most important part. If you don't take the time to prepare the walls, you will see bumps, cracks, and smudges after paint is applied. Just as in painting a room, when counseling with MI, significant preparation is needed before the client can begin to consider an action plan. Painting is the fun part. There's something wonderful about picking a color and seeing it come to life on the wall. The most important part though is preparing your walls so the paint glides on smoothly. Take the time to engage with the client, build rapport, and build motivation for change. Only when the client has expressed an earnest desire to make a change can the planning process ensue.

CHAPTER 5

Planning for Change

After all, when you seek advice from someone it's certainly not because you want them to give it. You just want them to be there while you talk to yourself.
—TERRY PRATCHETT

The fourth and final process of MI centers on developing a plan for change. The practitioner allows the client to take the lead in coming up with a change plan. If the client gets stuck, the practitioner can provide suggestions to help the client along. Once clients enter into planning, keep in mind it is not an invitation to start pelting them with unsolicited advice or information. In this chapter we'll consider ways to provide nutrition and fitness information without overstepping the client's autonomy in the change process.

INFORMATION EXCHANGE

Providing evidence-based information is an important part of nutrition and fitness counseling. In the spirit of MI, the practitioner acts as a guide and the client is the expert. The client is in charge of his body and behaviors and is given the respect to make his own decisions. However, you are there to help him brainstorm the best way to go about making the change or provide information about the latest research for a particular disease state, fitness plan, dietary supplement, or nutrient. During the action planning process, guide the client to consider multiple solutions for the behavior change. This may involve inviting him to come up with strategies, offering ideas that have worked for other people, asking him to devise goals, and troubleshooting the behavior change process.

When done at the right time with the right tactics, information sharing enriches the counseling experience for both the client and the practitioner. Below are some specific strategies for providing information in a way that keeps the client engaged as you navigate a behavior change plan together.

Asking Permission

Many nutrition and fitness practitioners fear they will not be able to tell their clients everything they need to hear in the time allotted. For some, this anxiety causes the practitioner to get to the point quickly and begin sharing information. We discourage the "get to the point" tactic, because it forces the client into a passive role. The benefits of motivational interviewing are apparent when clients take an active role, taking responsibility for making changes in their lives. To guide clients to take an active role, consider asking permission before giving any suggestions. Asking permission and respecting clients' answers puts them in the driver's seat.

> PRACTITIONER: You care about getting your blood sugars into a normal range and mentioned a desire to cut back on the amount of crackers you eat.
>
> CLIENT: Yes, I've been working at this for 15 years, but it seems like my diabetes has changed recently. So I can't keep doing the same thing. I need to change the way I do things.
>
> PRACTITIONER: How do you think you'll go about making this change?
>
> CLIENT: You know, that's where I'm stuck. I've been at this for so long, I'm not sure where to go from here.
>
> PRACTITIONER: I have some suggestions you might consider. Would you be interested in hearing them?
>
> CLIENT: Yes, that's what I'm here for.

It's important to note that if a client does not accept your request to give information, it is an indication that he isn't ready to consider what you have to say. It doesn't necessarily mean the client is unwilling to make any changes or take an active role in the behavior change process; it only means you may have misjudged the client's stage of change or missed earlier cues of sustain talk. It's also possible that you haven't spent enough time engaging the client, or that the client feels forced to select a particular behavior change that doesn't align with his interests.

The benefits of motivational interviewing are apparent when clients take an active role, taking responsibility for making changes in their lives.

It has been our experience that clients typically do not refuse suggestions outright. It is more likely that the client will agree to listen to your suggestions, but if unready to make a change, he may explain why each idea you provide will not work. If a client turns down your offer to provide strategies that might help him along in the behavior change process, or expresses disinterest in a wide variety of tips and ideas, back up and revisit the engaging, focusing, or evoking processes.

Elicit–Provide–Elicit

Elicit–provide–elicit (E-P-E), also known as explore–offer–explore (E-O-E), is a step-by-step model that outlines how to sandwich information provided to the client between two open-ended questions (see Figure 5.1).

Elicit

The practitioner first elicits or gathers information on what the client already knows about the nutrition or fitness topic. By finding out what the client already knows, you can learn about the client's stage of change and identify any signs of hesitation toward behavior change.

Most important, when you do give information you can spend your time building on what your client already knows, instead of boring him with details he doesn't need. In addition, the client may have misconceptions about the topic. Eliciting his or her current understanding can clue you in to opportunities to later correct misunderstandings, if needed. (For more information on clarifying misinformation, see Chapter 12.)

By first eliciting what the client already knows about a topic, you can assess the client's intellectual ability and communication style. In many

---

Elicit
- Ask the client what he already knows about the topic.
- Ask the client what else he'd like to know about the topic.
- Ask permission to provide information.

Provide
- Share only relevant information.
- Use the client's experiences as a starting point and assess what is already known.
- Keep it short and sweet.
- Avoid using imperatives, such as "You should" or "All you need to do is. . . ."

Elicit
- Check in with the client.
- Invite the client to respond to the information provided by asking a question such as, "What are your thoughts on that?."

FIGURE 5.1. Elicit–provide–elicit.

situations the client may feel uncomfortable if the educator uses language that is too advanced. If the client first verbalizes what he already knows about a topic or disease state, you can make sure to speak at the client's level of understanding.

In that same vein, you can also ask the client what else she would like to know about the nutrition or fitness topic before providing information. By assessing the client's knowledge gaps, you are sure to provide information that aligns with her interests and needs. This initial elicit also typically includes a permission question before providing the client with the information. The act of eliciting the client's current understanding and knowledge gaps while also asking permission before providing information honors the client's autonomy and demonstrates a desire to meet the client's needs.

Provide

As we suggested earlier, provide the information or strategies for change that build on what the client already knows or needs. During the provide stage, observe the client's verbal and nonverbal cues to determine whether the client is engaged, interested, and understands the facts given. It's important to offer information that is relevant, useful, and brief. When providing suggestions to clients, they will be more willing to consider what you've said if given more than one solution.

For example, if a practitioner were to offer practical strategies for increasing physical activity with a working mom, he might suggest taking the stairs at work, using alternative transportation, or walking during a lunch break. To strengthen client autonomy it can be helpful to follow up the list of options by saying, "It's up to you." By giving clients a menu of options and asking for their input, you will avoid situations where they leave the session feeling overwhelmed with food and exercise rules.

Elicit

After providing information, check in with the client to assess interest in and understanding of the ideas provided. The conversation reengages the client as you elicit further details about how the client feels or what she thinks of the information given. In this final elicit, open-ended questions are commonly used to check in with the client. Here are some examples:

"What do you think about these ideas?"
"How do you think this would work in your life?"
"Which of these ideas, if any, interest you?"

In the following example, the practitioner uses an E-P-E technique to provide the client with nutrition facts for end-stage renal failure with dialysis treatment. When the practitioner provides information, she gives a list of options from which the client can select. This dialogue begins in the middle of a session after the client has expressed change talk and appears ready to receive information.

> PRACTITIONER: You mentioned earlier that it's important for you to be able to be a part of your grandkids' lives.
>
> CLIENT: I just want to be an active part of their lives, not just a grandfather who sits back and watches everything.
>
> PRACTITIONER: You want to be in the game. What have you already heard about nutrition for dialysis? [elicit]
>
> CLIENT: Well, I remember my doctor saying I'm going to need to eat more protein, but I just hate those dialysis protein drinks.
>
> PRACTITIONER: You're right, increasing your protein will help to improve your overall health while on dialysis. There are many ways to increase your protein other than drinking supplements. Are you interested in hearing them? [asking permission]
>
> CLIENT: Sure.
>
> PRACTITIONER: Some dialysis patients eat more eggs, whereas others prefer beef, poultry, pork, or fish. [provide] In fact, I have a handout on high-protein meal ideas for individuals on dialysis. Would this be helpful for you?
>
> CLIENT: Yes. That would be great. My wife will appreciate it.
>
> PRACTITIONER: What are your thoughts on these ideas? [elicit]
>
> CLIENT: I think eating more meat is a much better way for me to get more protein.

Giving Advice

The client benefits most if the practitioner is in a trusted but equal position, and gives the client a sense of unconditional acceptance. Advice giving is discouraged in an MI session because it makes the client feel that you have all the answers. While you may in fact have many solutions that you believe can help your client move forward, your goal within an MI session is to support your client to develop his own action plan. You are there to clarify misinformation, offer suggestions, and guide the client to make meaningful and effective changes. Giving advice, especially without

While you may in fact have many solutions that you believe can help your client move forward, your goal within an MI session is to support your client to develop his own action plan.

asking permission first, will likely result in sustain talk, and possible discord within the counseling relationship, ultimately slowing the client's process toward change.

Even if the client asks you what he should do, he may not necessarily be ready to make changes. If he is in a contemplative or preparation stage of change it may be more helpful to respond by eliciting the client's own thoughts and feelings.

As in many aspects of MI, your choice of language during the planning process is important. Avoid using imperatives such as "What you need to do is . . . ," "You should just . . . ," or "What *you* want to do is. . . . " Whether the clients say it out loud or not, they will likely begin to argue with your point or share reasons why making that change isn't possible. Clients need to talk themselves into change, not the other way around.

Offering a Concern

There may be times when a client starts voicing change talk for a behavior change that you don't think is a good idea. Try to catch yourself before you say something like, "No, that's not what you want to do." Your role will be to help the client come to that conclusion on his own. Use reflective listening statements in a neutral tone of voice to gain understanding and evoke the client's reasons and feelings. This also may be the right time to offer a concern. By offering your concern for the client to consider, you allow him to remain the expert and make his own decision about what he'll ultimately do. For example, if a client is expressing interest in trying a very restrictive diet, it is appropriate for you to voice the reasons why it might not be a good idea. It is always the client's choice what to do; however, it is the practitioner's job to make sure the client has the right information to make a decision.

When offering a concern, be honest and open with the client without arguing. The client may be less likely to argue or react with sustain talk if you ask permission before offering your concern.

In the following example, the practitioner offers the client a concern she has about her interest in trying meal replacement shakes.

> CLIENT: I just need to drink those diet shakes for breakfast and lunch. Then, no matter what I have for dinner, I'll still lose weight. I've already gone to the store and bought a batch of them. They're really good.
>
> PRACTITIONER: You're excited to start making some positive changes in your eating patterns. [affirmation] What concerns do you have about how this might go? [open-ended question]

CLIENT: None, really. I've tried diets like this before and I seem to lose a lot of weight in a short amount of time. So it does work.

PRACTITIONER: You've noticed in the short term that you lose weight when sticking to a diet with meal replacement shakes. What was it about this eating plan that made you stop? [open-ended question]

CLIENT: I think I just wasn't motivated enough last time. I'm newly single and so I really need to lose this weight since I need to get out there and start dating again.

PRACTITIONER: You're anxious to start seeing some results. [reflection] However, I have a concern about the approach you've chosen. Can I share my concern with you? [asking permission]

CLIENT: Yes.

PRACTITIONER: I'm concerned that this dieting plan could be too restrictive. Researchers consistently show that weight-loss plans based on diet shakes help people lose weight in the short term but end with regaining the weight in the long run. Some of my clients have also experienced feelings of failure and body dissatisfaction following these types of plans. They often get tired of drinking the shakes over time. Of course, you're the expert on your body, so it's up to you what you choose to do. I just want to make sure you have all the information before you make your decision. What do you think about what I've just shared?

In this example the practitioner gives the client a chance first to consider any risks involved with the proposed behavior change. When the client does not mention any concerns, the practitioner shares what she knows based on the latest research. She does so by first asking permission. She offers the concern and then elicits a response from the client.

CLIENT-CENTERED GOAL SETTING

Within action planning, check in with the client and ask if there are specific goals he would like to make. In other words, what specific change is he interested in trying? Or perhaps there are certain thought patterns or beliefs he would like to explore on his own before the next appointment, like why he eats when he's not hungry or why he feels compelled to finish his plate although he's already full. There may even be a type of exploration activity or experiment that the client would like to attempt on his own. This is the client's opportunity to define personal goals, making them more specific, or just to repeat intentions to change.

Here are examples of realistic nutrition- and fitness-related goals that a client may set during a session with a nutrition or fitness practitioner:

- Sign up for a dance class.
- Add a cooked vegetable to dinner three nights a week.
- Eat more mindfully by turning off the TV off when eating dinner.
- Start packing a lunch to take to work.
- Provide a toddler with water instead of juice or soda between meals.
- Look for healthy crock pot recipes and try one.
- Fill out a food and feelings journal for 1 week like the one provided in Handout 5.1.

The client may select a specific goal or a more general one. Some people work best with numbers and timelines, while others may be reluctant under that type of pressure. Therefore, it is important that the client leads the goal-setting agenda. Clients will feel more empowered to follow through with a goal they select themselves than they would with a goal you give them. Some open-ended questions you can use to assist the client in the goal setting process include:

"Now that we've talked about all of the different options for how to go about making this change, is there any one specific part that you'd like to focus on?"

"Out of all of the things we've talked about, what specific change, if any, would you like to try?"

"What ideas do you have of specific changes you'd like to work on?"

"We've just discussed a little experiment you'd like to try. Are there any other experiments you would like to try after you leave here?"

"It sounds like you're not quite ready to make any changes at this point. I wonder if you would be interested in spending some time on your own brainstorming all the ways this change might affect your life and sharing what you come up with at our next appointment."

Below are two sample dialogues. In the first dialogue, the practitioner is guiding the goal setting. In the second example, the practitioner is allowing the client to lead the goal-setting process.

Practitioner-Led Goal Setting

PRACTITIONER: In your efforts to switch to a vegetarian diet, you mentioned a desire to add more protein-rich foods to your dinner meals. You said you liked beans. How about if we set a goal of including beans in a meal four nights a week?

Handout 5.1

FOOD AND FEELINGS JOURNAL

Use this journal to record your eating habits for a few days. By writing down your food and feelings you may become more aware of the reasons behind your food selection and how certain foods make your body feel. Start by noting the time of day and the foods you eat. Focus on the physical sensations before you eat and after you've finished. Write down any feelings that arise. An example is provided in the first row. This activity can help you identify times of the day, single foods, food combinations, or emotional triggers that motivate troublesome eating experiences.

Time	Food	How does your body feel before you eat?	How does your body feel after you eat?	Overall emotional feelings
9:00 a.m.	Cold fiber cereal with milk, cup of coffee with half and half, strawberries	Stomach is fluttering with hunger, but only barely.	Satisfied and content	Had to remind myself to slow down and pay attention to my food/how my body feels. Surprised when I left some cereal in the bowl, but I felt satisfied.

(continued)

Handout 5.1 (*continued*)

CLIENT: OK, sure, I can do that.

PRACTITIONER: Great! Here are some recipes that I think you'll like.

CLIENT: Yes, that bean and corn salad recipe sounds pretty easy to make.

PRACTITIONER: OK, so four nights a week you will include some sort of legume to your dinner meal. To be successful with this goal, you will need to get to the grocery store. Be sure to write the ingredients you need for your recipes on a list before you go.

CLIENT: Yes, I get lazy with shopping lists sometimes, so I will try to be better about that.

Client-Led Goal Setting

PRACTITIONER: In your efforts to switch over to a vegetarian diet, you mentioned a desire to add more protein-rich foods to your dinner meals. We've discussed a few ideas. Which ideas appeal to you the most?

CLIENT: I like the idea of adding beans to some of the meals I already make. I'm also interested in trying out some of the premade items you mentioned like vegetarian burgers and sausage. I don't have a lot of time to spend in the kitchen in the evenings and those ideas are the easiest.

PRACTITIONER: Given your time constraints and taste preferences, adding beans and frozen items are a good place to start. As you begin making this new change, is it helpful for you to have a goal in mind, in terms of a certain number of days per week to add these foods to your dinner meals?

CLIENT: Yes, I do better when I know exactly what I'm aiming for.

PRACTITIONER: What sounds like a reasonable goal to start with?

CLIENT: I should probably start small, like two days a week.

PRACTITIONER: OK, two days a week. What can I provide at this point to help you reach your goal?

CLIENT: I can't think of anything.

PRACTITIONER: What ideas do you have for specific meals that include the foods we've discussed?

CLIENT: I know I can make beans and rice, but I'm sure I can come up with other ideas.

PRACTITIONER: I have some vegetarian recipes here that include beans. Would you be interested in looking at those for some ideas?

CLIENT. Yes.

PRACTITIONER: Here they are. Which, if any, of these sound appealing?

CLIENT: I like that corn and bean salad recipe. I'm going to try that one this week.

PRACTITIONER: You sound ready to make this change. What other pieces of this protein-boost can I help you with?

CLIENT: Nothing. I think I can do this. I just need to make sure I've got the items I need on my grocery list. I get lazy with shopping lists sometimes, so I will try to be better about that.

PRACTITIONER: You sound excited to start adding protein-rich foods to your dinner meals two days a week. Would it be helpful to talk through the grocery shopping part before you go?

CLIENT: Yes, I guess I do need help with that part as well.

In the first dialogue, the practitioner pushes the client toward a specific goal without checking in with the client to see if it sounds feasible. In addition, the practitioner provides unsolicited advice and recipes without checking first to see whether the client needs the information. The cost of a practitioner-driven goal-setting process is that the practitioner may select a goal that is too challenging to meet, ultimately setting the client up to fail.

In the second dialogue, the practitioner kept checking in with the client, asking her first whether naming a specific goal is useful and then inviting the client to set a feasible goal. Once the goal was set, the practitioner didn't stop there, but continued to ask what additional information might be useful. Allowing the client to lead the goal-setting process supports client autonomy and gives the client confidence in setting personal health goals independently in the future.

If clients are truly in charge of selecting a specific goal or action, then they will likely come up with something they believe to be achievable and appropriate for their lives. However, there may be times when clients specify goals that seem unrealistic. You may be tempted to try to talk your clients out of a particular goal. It is important that they feel supported in the goal setting, no matter what they choose. As opposed to arguing with clients about setting more realistic goals, the practitioner can ask questions to explore any potential barriers to change or offer a concern, as discussed previously.

Setting Up an Experiment

When clients have trouble reaching unrealistic goals, they feel they have failed. The thought of embarking on a permanent lifestyle change can be overwhelming for some. You can make a behavior change less daunting for your client if you frame it as an experiment. By inviting a client to set up a temporary change, you give him the opportunity to try a certain behavior without making a lifelong commitment to it; it's like dipping a toe in the baby pool instead of jumping into the deep end. Through the trial run the client can find out whether he is capable of the change, whether he likes the change, and also how the change influences others around him.

Testing out behavior changes can also be helpful in guiding the client to visualize and reflect on it from many angles. As with any experiment, start by asking the client what factors she would like to pay attention to or notice as she attempts to make the change. This is like collecting data while performing a scientific experiment. If at the end of the experiment, the data collected by the client is positive, then the client may decide to make the change permanent. If the client finds that the change interfered significantly with other areas of life, then she may decide at her next appointment to select a different action item. If your client has trouble coming up with ideas of items to monitor as she's making the change, here are some suggestions:

- Her overall satisfaction with the meal.
- How she feels after dinner.
- What her energy level is like.
- What her fullness level reflects.
- Regularity of bowel movements.

At a follow-up visit, speak to the client about the results of the experiment with curiosity, not judgment. By maintaining an aura of curiosity, the client can safely reflect on the experience with a fresh perspective.

In the following dialogue, the practitioner guides the client to attempt a behavior change for the first time in the form of an experiment:

> PRACTITIONER: You said you'd like to stop eating before you're uncomfortably full. [reflection] How would you feel about testing out this behavior change this week, like an experiment? [open-ended question]
>
> CLIENT: Sounds fun, I guess. What kind of experiment?
>
> PRACTITIONER: Perhaps you'd like to pick a few meals next week where you sit at the table and make a conscious effort to eat slower. Then you could report back at your next appointment with what the experience was like. [information giving]
>
> CLIENT: Yes, that sounds like a good idea.
>
> PRACTITIONER: Which days might be best to try this? [close-ended question]

CLIENT: Any day but Friday. We go out with friends on Fridays and I know it will be much harder when I'm not at home. How about Monday, Tuesday, and Wednesday?

PRACTITIONER: You'd like to try out three different dinner meals on Monday, Tuesday, and Wednesday. [reflection] What might be useful to notice as you try this change? [open-ended question]

CLIENT: I'll be curious to see how long it takes me to eat the meal. I could also pay attention to how I feel afterward. If I overeat I have a hard time sleeping. I have a feeling I'll actually sleep better if I'm not feeling so bloated when I go to bed.

PRACTITIONER: So you'd like to think about the time it takes to finish a meal when you slow down, how you feel afterward, and how this change influences your sleep. [reflection] Anything else? [open-ended question]

CLIENT: I think that's pretty good. I think this change will really help.

The practitioner invited the client to set up an experiment and a specific goal. Once decided, the practitioner asked the client to monitor the outcomes of the experiment by asking, "What might be useful to notice as you try this change?" The client is leaving the practitioner's office with a game plan. She is going to test the waters of change through conducting a small experiment and assess whether the benefits of making the change are worth her efforts.

ASSESSING CONFIDENCE AND PERCEIVED BARRIERS TO CHANGE

A primary goal of a nutrition or fitness counseling session is to help clients increase confidence in making a behavior change. Therefore, it's a good idea to check in with them before they head home regarding their feelings about the action steps they plan to take. Through a short conversation at the end of a session, the client and practitioner can explore any potential barriers to change and take a look at the client's overall confidence in changing.

A simple scaling question, followed by probing questions and reflective listening, can help you assess a client's confidence. Perhaps there is some last-minute troubleshooting you can do to assist the client in the change. The following example includes a scaling question to assess confidence, followed by a series of questions to assess barriers and develop strategies to overcome those barriers.

PRACTITIONER: You've mentioned an interest in trying to include an afternoon snack each workday. How confident are you on a scale from 0 to 10 that you can make this change, with 0 being not at all confident and 10 being very confident? [scaling question]

CLIENT: I'm at about 7.

PRACTITIONER: Tell me about your answer. Why not an 8 or a 6? [open-ended question]

CLIENT: Well, I'm hungry in the afternoon, so I'm sure I'll remember to eat. I'm just not sure I'll remember to pack my afternoon snack, so I may end up eating something out of the vending machine instead. I'm not sure I'll feel good about that.

PRACTITIONER: So you're fairly confident that you'll be able to eat an afternoon snack most days, but you're not as confident that you'll be eating a healthy snack. [reflection]

CLIENT: Right.

PRACTITIONER: What do you think will get in the way of packing and bringing that snack with you to work? [open-ended question]

CLIENT: I think it's just a memory issue. I'm afraid I'll forget.

PRACTITIONER: What might help you remember? [open-ended question]

CLIENT: I could probably put a reminder on my phone that goes off 10 minutes before I leave the house.

PRACTITIONER: And you think that this type of alarm reminder might do the trick. [reflection]

CLIENT: Yeah, it's the only way I remember anything.

Nutrition and fitness practitioners often skip client-driven goal setting because they are short on time, or confident that the counseling techniques used were sufficient to ensure client success. However, if you take a few extra minutes at the end of the appointment to check in with the client, he may feel a little more confident leaving your office.

> *Remember that motivation is based on factors such as a client's ability, confidence, and belief that efforts to change will work.*

The acronym GAB is a useful memory technique to remember the final conversation before the client leaves the office. Before the client heads out the door, "GAB" with him for a few minutes:

Goals: Invite the client to share one last time what behavior or thought pattern he will attempt to change.

Assess confidence: Use a scaling question to assess the client's confidence in his ability to make the proposed behavior change or thought pattern.

Barriers: Invite the client to consider any potential barriers that may get in his way and strategies to overcome them (if any).

It's exciting when clients get to the point where they are ready to start making changes. You hear them start to talk about the future in a positive way, voicing mobilizing change talk such as commitment, activation, and steps they'll take to achieve their goals. Remember that motivation is based on factors such as a client's ability, confidence, and belief that efforts to change will work. Although the client may seem ready, there are reasons why he or she hasn't already made the change. Check in with clients to assess their confidence, troubleshoot their barriers, and provide relevant information when necessary. The action-planning process can be a rewarding time for both the client and the practitioner, as clients gain new strategies to test the waters of change.

PART III

Mastering the Microskills: OARS

CHAPTER 6

Open-Ended Questions

The greatest compliment that was ever paid me was when one asked me what I thought, and attended to my answer.
—HENRY DAVID THOREAU

Questions are a customary component of conversation. The word *interviewing* in the term *motivational interviewing* suggests the important role questions play in evoking motivation from a client. By asking questions, the practitioner expresses interest in understanding the client. In the spirit of MI, the client is the expert of her life. Therefore, questions are used to elicit her expertise, thereby putting her in the driver's seat of the change-making process. While a variety of different types of questions are used in a typical motivational interviewing session, the most important questions are those that evoke change talk. Asking questions is just one key skill commonly used in MI.

The four microskills of MI are:

1. **O**pen-ended questions
2. **A**ffirmations
3. **R**eflections
4. **S**ummaries

Together, they are known as OARS. Much of what the practitioner says during an MI session falls into one of these four categories. The primary purpose of using OARS is to elicit and emphasize the client's change talk through reflective listening strategies, while attending for opportunities to affirm the client in his or her quest toward making a behavior change.

OARS will be covered in detail in this section of the book, with a chapter on each concept. This chapter includes strategies for formulating open-ended questions that evoke change talk and encourage your clients to come up with solutions for changing nutrition and fitness behaviors.

OPEN-ENDED VERSUS CLOSED-ENDED QUESTIONS

Open-ended questions are worded in such a way as to elicit a meaningful and thoughtful response from the client. Conversely, closed-ended questions are those that elicit only a single word or a nondescriptive phrase. Open-ended questions are preferred over closed-ended questions as they encourage the client to give voice to their thoughts, feelings, experiences, opinions, values, and motivations (see Figure 6.1). The following are examples of open-ended questions:

"What brings you here today?"
"What troubles you about this way of eating?"
"How have you dealt with that in the past?"
"How do you think this way of eating is affecting your health or well-being?"

In contrast, a closed question, although necessary at times, tends to limit the client's response. Examples of closed-ended questions include:

"Do you like running?"
"How many times do you plan on doing this each week?"
"What is your height?"
"Which days of the week did you try this change?"
"Do you prefer weekdays or weekend days?"
"Do you like fruits and vegetables?"

Open-ended questions are more likely to evoke change talk than closed-ended questions. Therefore, aim to ask open-ended questions at least 70% of the time. While this concept makes sense conceptually, it can be challenging to carry out. The payoff is well worth mastering this technique. When the practitioner chooses just the right evocative open-ended question, the client can begin to process barriers and motivators to change. Now and then a close-ended question may be the only option. For example, MI practitioners often ask closed-ended questions such as, "Is it all right if I show you some different topics we could discuss today?" or "Would you like to schedule a follow-up session?" However, in general, open-ended questions are best for building a relationship with your client.

FORMING AN OPEN-ENDED QUESTION

To turn a closed question into an open-ended question, it may help to use a sentence starter such as *how*, *what*, *why*, or *tell me*. Although a sentence starting with "Tell me" is not technically a question, it is a good way to encourage the client to elaborate on what was previously said, thereby

Open-ended questions are typically started with the following words or phrases:
"How . . . ?"
"What . . . ?"
"Why . . . ?"*
"Tell me. . . . "
Use caution when starting a sentence with why. It can easily be perceived as judgmental.
Closed-ended questions are typically started with the following words or phrases:
"Do you . . . ?"
"Have you . . . ?"
"Are you . . . ?"
"Will you . . . ?"
"Is it . . . ?"
"Can you . . . ?"

FIGURE 6.1. Starting an open-ended question.

serving as an open-ended question. For example, if you say, "Tell me what that was like," you will likely receive an in-depth response that gives you clues into the way your client processes experiences.

While "why" questions are open-ended, they come with caution tape. The practitioner can easily come off as condescending or judgmental. The following "why" questions reduce autonomy and result in the client feeling pressured to change:

"Why don't you want to do it?"
"Why can't you?"
"Why haven't you?"
"Why do you need to?"
"Why don't you . . . ?"

It may be best to avoid these types of questions altogether. If "why" questions are used, be mindful of your tone of voice to minimize sounding judgmental. Figure 6.2 illustrates how closed-ended questions can be transformed into open-ended questions to encourage clients to elaborate.

BENEFITS OF OPEN-ENDED QUESTIONS

There are many benefits to using open-ended questions. Here are just a few:

- *Talk therapy.* The simple act of talking can be therapeutic for some clients. Talking through struggles surrounding food and activity to a kind and listening ear can reduce stress and anxiety.

Closed-ended question	Open-ended question
• "Do you have any concerns about your current level of physical activity?"	• "What concerns, if any, do you have about your current level of physical activity?"
• "Do you want to go to our diabetes class?"	• "How would you feel about attending a diabetes class?"
• "Can you tell me more about that?"	• "Tell me more about that."
• "Do you like whole-grain bread?"	• "What's your opinion of whole-grain bread?"
• "How many days a week do you currently go to the gym?"	• "Describe your gym patterns."
• "What is your weight?"	• "Tell me about your weight or dieting history."
• "Do you want to be here?"	• "How do you feel about being here?"
• "Do you want to change the way you eat?"	• "What interest, if any, do you have in making a change in your eating habits?"
• "Can you think of any reasons for making this change?"	• "What are your reasons for making this change?"
• "Are there any barriers to making this change?"	• "What barriers, if any, will there be to making this change?"

FIGURE 6.2. Turning closed-ended questions into open-ended questions.

• *Ah-ha moments.* The right open-ended question at the right time can result in an "ah-ha" moment for the client. Through certain evoking types of open-ended questions, the practitioner is inviting the client to think about personal thoughts, feelings, and values. Often, through voicing out loud what the client is experiencing, he or she may find that a lightbulb clicks on and suddenly there is a sense of understanding or resolve.

• *Enhances reflective listening.* Reflective listening is a key skill in motivational interviewing that demonstrates empathy and builds trust. If clients are only responding to closed-ended questions with one word or a phrase, then the practitioner has little to reflect. However, when the practitioner asks open-ended questions and the client elaborates, there is more for the practitioner to reflect and highlight for the client to hear.

• *Minimizes leading questions.* Closed-ended questions lead the client into a certain response. For example, "How many servings of vegetables do you eat in a day?" is a leading question because the client may feel uncomfortable admitting he does not eat any vegetables. Thus, it is implied that there is a right and a wrong answer. An open-ended question that may better yield a truthful and more meaningful response would be "What are your eating habits like?"

• *Demonstrates interest and respect.* Open-ended questions tell the client that you value all that he has to say. Coupled with reflections, the client begins to feel that you understand him and have a genuine interest in his welfare.

• *Elicits change talk.* Perhaps the most important benefit of open-ended questions is the potential for eliciting change talk. Since the amount of change talk in a session predicts client success in making a change (Gaume, Bertholet, Faouzi, Gmel, & Daeppen, 2013; Barnett et al., 2014; Vader, Walters, Prabhu, Houck, & Field, 2010), it is important to ask questions that result in change talk.

> *Open-ended questions tell the client that you value all that he has to say. Coupled with reflections, the client begins to feel that you understand him and have a genuine interest in his welfare.*

OPEN-ENDED QUESTIONS: TOO MUCH OF A GOOD THING?

Questions are just one of the microskills of motivational interviewing. Overusing questions can lead to the question–answer trap (see Chapter 10). When a client is peppered with question after question, she may feel that the practitioner is either not listening or has taken the role of the expert within the appointment. To avoid rapid-fire questioning, aim to use reflections and open-ended questions in a 2:1 ratio—two reflections for every open-ended question. Notice how the practitioner alternates between reflections and open-ended questions in the dialogue below.

PRACTITIONER: What concerns, if any, do you have about your blood sugar being high? [open-ended question]

CLIENT: Well, I know it's not good.

PRACTITIONER: You've heard there are some health consequences to high blood sugar. [reflection]

CLIENT: Yes, like I remember my mom had terrible trouble with pain in her feet. Oh, it was awful.

PRACTITIONER: You've seen first-hand what can happen and you don't want to go through what your mom did. [reflection] What other things concern you? [open-ended question]

Notice that before the practitioner asks another question, he reflects the client's answer. Remembering to reflect after most client responses is a good way to ensure you will avoid the question–answer trap. Clients will feel heard and appreciated, which will likely result in additional sharing.

Practitioners often feel that knowledge is power; the more known about the client, the better. While it is true that certain pieces of information about a client are essential, too much focus on assessment can hinder the client–counselor relationship. Drilling the client with assessment-based questions places the expert hat on the practitioner and sends the client into a passive role, often responding with short, simple answers. A collaborative partnership can be easily dismantled in this type of Q-and-A dialogue.

A collaborative partnership can be easily dismantled in this type of Q-and-A dialogue.

Firing assessment questions one after another could backfire, leaving the client feeling defensive and less likely to elaborate. A number of strategies can be used to allow for assessment data collection while still maintaining engagement with the client. Consider the following options:

• *Engage before assessing.* Take plenty of time to build rapport with the client prior to conducting an oral assessment. Miller and Rollnick (2013) recommend refraining from asking assessment questions for the first 10 minutes of a session. Often, during the engagement process the counselor finds out a great deal about the client. The client may inadvertently answer many of the typical assessment questions during the dialogue that occurs naturally at the beginning of a session.

• *Limit the number of assessment questions.* Given all of the topics recommended within a complete nutritional assessment, as part of the NCP, an entire appointment could potentially be spent on assessment alone. As a practitioner, it's important to consider how much assessment is essential. For example, consider a complete dietary recall. Dietitians and nutritionists are trained to obtain an accurate dietary recall by asking specific questions regarding types of food, cooking methods, and exact amounts. In some cases, this information may be needed and in other cases, gaining this information will not change the focus of the counseling session. At times, certain assessment questions are mandated and may be unavoidable. When this is the case, it may be useful to ask clients to answer those questions on a clipboard in the waiting room prior to being seen.

• *Preappointment questionnaire.* Some practitioners prefer to use a preappointment questionnaire. By asking the client to answer assessment questions prior to a counseling session, more of the appointment can be spent addressing the client's specific needs. Some counselors ask the client to complete the questionnaire in the waiting room prior to the session and others send the questionnaire to the client via mail or email and ask the client to fill it out and send it in before the first session. If this method is used, the counselor may have a better sense of the client's primary concerns prior to the first visit and may be less likely to excessively question the client at the beginning of the appointment.

• *Maintain OARS throughout assessment.* Another strategy for maintaining engagement while collecting assessment data is to use open-ended questions, affirmations, reflections, and summaries. This often involves redesigning the counselor's list of assessment questions to limit closed-ended questions. For example, instead of asking for recent weight changes, consider an open-ended question like, "Tell me about your weight history." In addition, counselors can demonstrate active listening through providing accurate reflections and summaries, turning an oral assessment into a casual conversation.

TYPES OF OPEN-ENDED QUESTIONS

There are many different styles of open-ended questions and each has a place within an MI session.

Digging Deep

A lot of issues surrounding food are not about food. Behaviors are products of one's beliefs and values. Therefore, it's important to dig a little deeper to determine what else may be going on that's influencing behaviors and habits. The term *digging deep*, sometimes referred to as *unpacking*, is necessary when a client makes a statement and you suspect there may be more to the story. In other words, you may need to spend some time probing to uncover pertinent information about the client's situation, feelings, and reactions.

> A lot of issues surrounding food are not about food. Behaviors are products of one's beliefs and values.

There are three main reasons to dig deep with the client.

1. *Builds rapport.* By taking the time to dig deeper, you express to the client that he matters. These probing questions show that you are not only listening, but want to understand. In doing so, you build a stronger connection with the client.
2. *Enhances understanding.* Through listening to the client's answers to the probing questions, you can make sense of the issue at hand.
3. *Enhances client awareness.* In hearing himself talk about the issue, the client becomes more aware of his feelings and beliefs related to food and behavior change.

Statements that warrant digging a little deeper include:

"My husband has never had a weight problem, so he can eat whatever
  he wants."
"My mom does not understand how hard it is for me to lose weight."
"I am not a vegetable person."
"Certain foods make me sick."
"I should really cook at home more."
"I know I should just keep chocolate out of the house, or I'll eat all of
  it at once."
"I can't control myself around carbohydrates."
"I know I shouldn't eat after 7 P.M."

When you hear these one-liners and you get the feeling that there's
more to the story, hold back from immediately probing with additional
questions. First, provide a reflection to the client's statement to ensure that
you understand the meaning of what was said. These reflections can be
followed by open-ended questions to further explore the client's meaning.
Questions that can be used to dig deeper include:

"Tell me more about that."
"What's that like for you?"
"How so?"
"How does that make you feel?"
"Where do you think that idea came from?"
"What else?"
"What about that is important to you?"
"What is it about . . . that concerns you?"

Take the time needed to fully understand where the client is coming from. Individuals often have complicated feelings about food, fitness,
and body image. Slow down and encourage the client to explore underlying issues. In doing so, the client may experience an "ah-ha" moment or
uncover reasons behind a particular behavioral pattern.

In the following dialogue, a practitioner uses reflective listening followed by a "Tell me more" to unpack the client's personal meaning of the
word *binge*:

CLIENT: I can't even keep chocolate chip cookies in the house.

PRACTITIONER: You feel out of control around them.

CLIENT: Yes, especially when they are fresh out of the oven. I'll binge.

PRACTITIONER: You eat more than you'd like to and feel guilty after-
    ward.

CLIENT: Yes.

PRACTITIONER: You used the term *binge*. Tell me more about how you qualify a binge.

CLIENT: For cookies, I think four is too many.

PRACTITIONER: OK, for you, eating four cookies results in feelings of guilt afterward.

CLIENT: Yes, exactly.

"If Any" Questions

One way to express a nonjudgmental attitude is to avoid asking questions based on assumptions. Consider the question, "What concerns do you have about your high blood sugars?" Although this example is an open-ended question, it assumes the client is actually concerned about having high blood sugar. To make it less leading and judgmental, try making it an "if any" open-ended question. For example, tweak the question to: "What concerns, if any, do you have about your high blood sugars?" By qualifying a question with "if any" the practitioner gives the client a broad surface to work with, thereby enhancing autonomy. Asking a question based on an assumption can be risky because if the assumption is wrong the client may feel trapped and become defensive or shut down. By simply adding "if any," you give the client freedom to answer in any way. Here are other examples of "if any" questions:

> "What changes, if any, are you interested in making?"
> "Which of these topics, if any, are you interested in discussing today?"
> "What barriers, if any, might you run into?"

Change in the Abstract (Hypothetical Questions)

Another type of question is the hypothetical open-ended question: "If you made a change in this part of your life, how might it benefit you?" The hypothetical question gets the client to "try on" the idea and allows him or her to brainstorm through the potential barriers and the pros and cons. Here are other hypothetical questions:

> "If you were to attempt to cut back on soda in the next month, how would you go about doing it?"
> "If you were to talk to your spouse about needing his support for this change, what would you say?"
> "If you started packing a lunch next week, what foods would you need to buy first?"
> "If you started exercising this week, what activities might you try?"

Strengths-Based Questions

Self-efficacy, or the belief in one's ability under certain circumstances, is one of the cornerstones in building motivation. If a client understands what must be done but has no confidence in his abilities to implement these necessary changes, not much else will help. People with low self-efficacy tend to believe tasks are more difficult than those with higher self-efficacy. Guiding the client to talk about his strengths, skills, and accomplishments in related situations will help build self-efficacy moving the client one step closer toward making a behavior change.

The following questions are known as strengths-based questions because they invite the client to reflect on previous successes in similar situations:

> "What personal strengths have made you successful in making changes in the past?"
> "What's helped so far in managing your nutrition?"
> "What are you currently doing to manage stress in your life?"
> "What are the main things you're doing to support your overall health and well-being?"
> "Describe a time in the past when you were successful making a change. What was that like?"

A strengths-based question is particularly effective if followed by a statement affirming the characteristic outlined in the client's answer, as in the following dialogue:

> PRACTITIONER: What have been your successes, if any, since our last conversation? [open-ended question]
>
> CLIENT: Oh, I can't wait to tell you about last week. I thought about what we talked about and ended up cooking four nights last week.
>
> PRACTITIONER: When you put your mind to something, you do it. [affirmation]
>
> CLIENT: Well it was important to me. If only to show that I could do it.
>
> PRACTITIONER: You wanted to prove to yourself that you were capable of taking control of what you eat. [reflection]
>
> CLIENT: Yes, there's so much garbage out there; I'm just so tired of all the processed food and the way it makes me feel.
>
> PRACTITIONER: You noticed you feel better when you cook more at home. [reflection] What was it that made the difference in you reaching your goal last week? [open-ended question]

By using strengths-based questions, you can easily focus the client on acknowledging the positive physical or mental changes being made or that were made in the past. This technique is especially useful with clients who focus on why they can't make changes. If a client comes across as victimized, or failing to take responsibility for her actions, encourage her to talk about what she has done in the past to support her health.

Exploring Goals and Values

Everyone has specific goals, values, and priorities. By asking the client to share personal goals and values, you invite him to consider what he cares most about and examine how his values line up (or don't line up) with his actions and life choices.

Eating behavior is commonly connected with deeply held beliefs and values. Clients who abhor waste, for example, may find themselves consistently eating more than their bodies need in an attempt to avoid throwing away extra food. Examining this belief can help clients confront conflicting values. They are then free to decide how to change their behavior to accommodate their beliefs, or decide whether their belief is something they want to hold on to or discard.

Often there is discrepancy between a client's values and lifestyle choices. For example, a client may say that he values good health and has a goal of preventing a second heart attack. He may also mention that he hasn't been exercising at all in the last month. By asking a well-formed open-ended question to find out what's important to your client, you can invite him to explore possible discrepancies between goals, values, and behavior.

When asking these types of questions, it's important to do so without judgment. The client will likely notice the discrepancy himself, if asked in the right way. Here are some examples of questions that elicit discussion regarding goals and values:

"What do you value in your life?"
"How does your desire to improve your fitness line up with your values?"
"How do you like to prioritize your time on the weekends?"
"What do you care most about in life?"
"How does this change fit in with your personal values?"
"How do your current food and fitness choices align with your values?"

Reasons for Change

By inviting the client to express personal reasons for change, change talk will likely occur. These questions are essential in an MI session. By inviting the client to voice reasons for change, and then reflecting back those reasons, you help the client become aware and conscious of personal motivations for change. Here are examples of questions that almost always evoke change talk:

"Why do you want to change?"
"Why is now a good time to work on this?"
"What are some possible advantages to . . . ?"
"How could making this change make your life better?"
"How are your current ways of doing things not working for you?"

Looking Forward

Another way to elicit change talk is to invite the client to consider a future where the behavior change has been made, or to consider a future where the behavior change has not been made. These questions encourage the client to visualize possible long term benefits of change. Here are examples:

"If you decided to make this change, how would your life be different in the future?"
"When you look ahead 5 years of being successful with this change, how might your life be different?"
"Suppose you decide not to make this change. What might your life be like 5 years from now?"

Looking Back

Looking-back questions can also be effective in eliciting change talk. A looking-back question invites clients to consider a time when they were successful in making a change or life was generally better. In doing so, clients can compare these instances to the present to determine differences in attitudes and behaviors. Examples of looking-back questions include:

"Think back to a time when you didn't struggle with your body image. What was that like?"
"Was there ever a time when you didn't feel this way about food? How was life different back then?"
"Think back to a time in your life when you were more physically active. What was that like?"
"How do your current thoughts and feelings about your health compare to how you felt about it in the past?"

Often, in inviting the client to look back, she revisits a time before a problem arose. On occasion, doing so will result in the client revisiting a time when things were actually worse. If that's the case, you can guide the client to explore how she has actually improved over time, which may lead to a strengths-based question or affirmation.

Querying Extremes

Another way to elicit change talk is to invite clients to explore the best consequences of making the change and/or the worse consequences of not making the change. Doing so invites the client to consider best and worst case scenarios. Here are some examples:

> "What's most important to you about making this change?"
> "What's the best thing that could happen if you made this change?"
> "What concerns you most about your new diagnosis?"
> "Suppose you continued on without making any changes. What's the worst case scenario?"

Disarming Questions

Disarming questions invite the client to explore the reasons not to change. Clients may not be expecting this type of question. For example, a practitioner might ask, "What do you like about [current unchanged behavior]?" Disarming questions usually produce sustain talk. Therefore, it's important to use these questions minimally. When done right, disarming questions can alleviate resistance. At times, clients may even talk themselves into changing. Here are examples of disarming questions:

> "What do you like about binging?"
> "What do you like about eating at night in front of the TV?"
> "What do you like about the weeks when you're not active?"
> "There are important reasons that you haven't already made this change. What are those?"

It is important to note that these types of questions require an incredibly nonjudgmental tone from the practitioner. Any hint of sarcasm or judgment may result in discord.

Change Rulers

Using a change ruler is a great way to assess client's readiness, importance, interest, and confidence in change. A ruler question is one that asks the client to rate feelings about change on a scale, typically 0 to 10: "On a scale from 0 to 10 with 0 being not at all important and 10 being very important, how important is it to you to improve your energy by eating more regularly throughout the day?" Examples of change ruler questions include:

"How ready are you . . . ?"
"How important is it to you to . . . ?"
"How committed are you . . . ?"
"How confident are you . . . ?"
"How interested are you in . . . ?"
"How motivated are you . . . ?"

While the initial change ruler question is technically closed-ended, it's the open-ended follow-up questions that are essential in eliciting change talk. After the client shares a number, find out more about why the client selected that number. Probing questions that typically follow change ruler questions include:

"Tell me more about your answer."
"I noticed you didn't pick a lower number. Tell me about that." (This question typically produces change talk.)
"I noticed you didn't pick a higher number. Tell me about that." (This question typically produces sustain talk.)
"What could we talk about today that might increase your number?"

Some practitioners find it useful to keep a list of open-ended, evocative questions handy at each appointment that tend to be helpful during most sessions. Of course, the questions you choose to ask will ultimately depend on what you hear from your client. Figure 6.3 provides a sample list of evocative questions.

Putting It All Together

The following dialogue includes many different types of open-ended questions to evoke change talk.

> PRACTITIONER: What are your plans for feeding your infant after she's born? [open-ended question]
>
> CLIENT: I haven't decided yet. I'll probably bottle feed since it's easiest.
>
> PRACTITIONER: At this point, bottle feeding seems like an easier choice. [reflection] What is it about bottle feeding that seems like the easiest choice? [disarming open-ended question]
>
> CLIENT: Well, that way I can sort of pass the baby around to my mom and other people in my family for feedings. Then the responsibility won't always be on me.
>
> PRACTITIONER: You're hoping others will help out, and bottle feeding seems like the best way others might be able to help you. [reflection]

- "What was it like to receive that diagnosis?"
- "What matters most about it?"
- "What are the best and worst parts?"
- "What is important to you about this change? What does it mean to you?"
- "How important is it on a scale of 0 to 10?"
- "How motivated are you on a scale from 0 to 10 to . . . ?"
- "What would have to be different for the importance to be higher?"
- "How would your life be different after this change?"
- "How might this particular change get you what you want?"
- "How does this change relate to your personal values in life?"
- "What concerns do you have about what you are doing now? What bothers you most about it?"
- "What is good/working about what you do now?"
- "How might changing make your life worse?"
- "Who in your life would like this change?"
- "Who in your life would not like this change?"
- "How might others be able to support you in making this change?"
- "How is what you're doing right now not working for you?"
- "How would your life be different if you did decide to make changes?"
- "How would changing make your life better?"

FIGURE 6.3. Open-ended questions cheat sheet.

CLIENT: Yes. That way my boyfriend can get up in the middle of the night to feed her and I can keep sleeping.

PRACTITIONER: Bottle feeding in the middle of the night sounds easier to you. I also heard you say that you haven't completely decided yet. [summary] What is it about breastfeeding that has you on the fence? [reasons for change open-ended question]

CLIENT: I know that it will be a hassle to actually prepare the bottle in the middle of the night. Plus, I don't want to buy formula all the time.

PRACTITIONER: Fumbling around in the dark with bottles and formula isn't your idea of a good time. [reflection]

PRACTITIONER: At this point, how interested are you in breastfeeding on a scale from 0 to 10, with 10 being very interested and 0 being not at all interested? [change ruler]

CLIENT: I'd say that I'm at about a 6.

PRACTITIONER: You're on the fence about this. [reflection] Tell me why you chose a 6. [probing question]

CLIENT: Well, I'm worried I'm going to want to go out with my friends or something and not feel like I can leave my baby if I breastfeed. But my friends were telling me that breastfeeding would help me lose the baby weight.

PRACTITIONER: You're feeling conflicted. On one hand, you want to be able to continue to do the things you enjoy and on the other hand the benefit of weight loss following your pregnancy is a big motivator for you to breastfeed. [reflection]

CLIENT: Yeah, and I'm sure you're gonna tell me about how it's good for my baby too.

PRACTITIONER: You already know about some of the health benefits for your baby. [reflection] What have you heard? [reasons for change open-ended question]

CLIENT: I don't really know the details, I've just heard it's better for the baby.

PRACTITIONER: Would you like to hear more about that? [closed-ended ask permission question]

CLIENT: Not really. I don't need to know the details.

PRACTITIONER: All right. Let's see if I got it all. You're on the fence about breastfeeding, with your biggest concern being sharing the load of the feeding and having the flexibility to go out with your friends. You mentioned weight loss, your baby's health, saving money, and ease of feeding in the middle of the night as aspects that are important to you. You've also said you'd really like help from friends and family. Perhaps you're wondering if you breast-fed, how they might help take care of the baby so that you could get more sleep. [summary]

CLIENT: Lord knows I'm going to need some help!

PRACTITIONER: If you were to breastfeed, what are some ways your friends and family could help you? [change in the abstract open-ended question]

CLIENT: I'm going to need babysitters so I can nap. I'm sure there will be diapers that will need changing!

PRACTITIONER: Right, so just being present during the day would be helpful. [reflection] Would you be interested in hearing other ways your friends and family could help if you did decide to breastfeed? [closed-ended, ask permission question]

CLIENT: Sure.

PRACTITIONER: They can help by burping the baby after feedings, doing laundry, and a breastfeeding mother needs more food, so perhaps you can put your loved ones to work in the kitchen cooking you meals and cleaning up afterward. [giving information] What do you think about those ideas? [open-ended question]

CLIENT: I like the sound of that!

Open-ended questions are a pivotal skill in building motivation for change. Well-placed open-ended questions guide the client to consider motivations, values, barriers, skills, and reasoning not previously considered. Open-ended questions along with affirmations, reflective listening statements, and summaries make up the essential skills of a productive and effective nutrition or fitness counseling session.

CHAPTER 7

Affirmations

A person who feels appreciated will always do more than what is expected.

—UNKNOWN

So encourage each other and build each other up, just as you are already doing.

—1 THESSALONIANS 5:11 (NLT)

Clients often have the skills and education required to start making changes. What they lack, however, is confidence in their ability to execute and sustain a specific behavior change. This belief in one's ability to change is known as *self-efficacy*. Clients may come to you having tried many different ways to change their eating and exercise patterns. Unfortunately, it is common that they come to you only after feeling the harsh reality of many failures. If nothing else, what these clients need is a boost in confidence. This chapter discusses the use of affirmations, or positive statements regarding one's character or values that ultimately result in strengthening self-efficacy, building rapport, and fueling change talk.

AFFIRMATIONS DEFINED

MI uses many techniques to build and support self-efficacy, but none so much as the strategic use of affirmations. An *affirmation* is a positive statement regarding one's character or values that acknowledges his or her strengths and efforts (Miller & Rollnick, 2013). The following statements are examples of positive affirmations:

"You are the type of person who works hard for what you have."
"You really care about people."

"You want to spare people the pain you've been through."
"You've really come to know what your body needs."
"It's important to you to be a good role model for your kids."
"You've learned to trust yourself when you're around sweets."
"It can be hard to face certain problems. Coming here took courage."
"You stuck to your goal even when it was challenging to do so."
"You have a lot of compassion in your heart."
"You know you can do it because you've done it before."

Affirmations can be simple sentences like the ones above or they can be found in the form of reframing reflections and summaries. When you highlight the positive components of a client's statement, you create an atmosphere of opportunity, unconditional positive regard, and support that permeates the entire encounter.

The opposite of an affirmation would be a negative statement or bias about the client. The idea that people will change if you make them feel bad about their bodies, eating habits, or physical activity patterns is problematic, and in fact the opposite appears to be true. When overweight and obese individuals feel discriminated against based on their weight they are more likely to gain weight (Sutin & Terracciano, 2013). On the other hand, people are more successful with change when they feel good about themselves.

The tendency to affirm is found in the practitioner's mindset. Constantly look for what clients do right, what they've accomplished, and how they are capable of realizing their goals. Changing your mindset to focus on, search for, and reflect the positive might sound a bit tiresome. However, with time and practice, it becomes a way of life.

> *When you highlight the positive components of a client's statement, you create an atmosphere of opportunity, unconditional positive regard, and support that permeates the entire encounter.*

BENEFITS OF AFFIRMATIONS

Affirmations help clients recognize their strengths and capabilities. A well-placed affirmation can lead to change talk by drawing the client's attention to the resources available within. In addition to supporting client self-efficacy, affirmations can help build a strong rapport between practitioner and client, boosting engagement. Affirmations benefit clients in a variety of ways. See Figure 7.1 for a list of 10 reasons to affirm your client.

In short, affirmations empower your client, encourage persistence and reduce discord. These three key benefits of affirming clients are expanded upon with examples below.

1. Empowers the client to believe in him- or herself in a specific area.
2. The client begins to internalize positive attributes.
3. Boosts overall self-confidence.
4. Encourages persistence.
5. Decreases defensiveness.
6. Opens people up to considering discrepancies and the possibility of change.
7. Strengthens or helps to repair the client–practitioner relationship.
8. The client feels supported.
9. Creates an atmosphere of positivity.
10. Supports forward momentum toward change.

FIGURE 7.1. Top 10 reasons to affirm your client.

Affirmations Empower the Client

In order to develop a well-constructed affirmation, the practitioner must not only listen but also make some assumptions about the meaning within the client's statements. There may be many opportunities throughout a counseling session to reframe a client statement to highlight positive characteristics. When a client feels confident in his or her abilities and focuses less on the barriers, the client can begin to consider change. Here is an example of an affirmation aimed at empowering the client.

CLIENT: I know I don't eat enough vegetables. When my sister was on [a commercial weight loss program] she was eating vegetables all the time.

PRACTITIONER: You saw your sister succeeding and you think it would work for you too. [reflection]

CLIENT: I guess so.

PRACTITIONER: If you did decide to add more vegetables to your diet, how would you go about it? [open-ended question]

CLIENT: I don't know. I've never done much with them before.

PRACTITIONER: You're a little unsure about how to prepare them and incorporate them into your meals and snacks. [reflection]

CLIENT: My sister has me over for dinner sometimes. One time she made a stir fry that I really liked. I guess I could ask her how she does it.

PRACTITIONER: You're not afraid to ask for help. And you're even willing to move out of your comfort zone and learn and try new things. [affirmation]

CLIENT: Only when I have a good teacher. I bet it would be better if I helped her make it one night.

Affirmations Encourage Persistence

Affirmations are helpful in directing clients in a positive direction. Here is an example using an affirmation to encourage persistence. A client with HIV is seeing a nutritionist to aid in preventing symptoms of malnutrition.

> CLIENT: Thinking about what and when to eat is a constant stress and some days I'm just too tired. [sustain talk]
>
> PRACTITIONER: You've been through a lot, and some days it wears you down; you're here today because you're not ready to give up. [reflection and affirmation]
>
> CLIENT: I can't give up. I have to do this. [change talk]
>
> PRACTITIONER: Tell me more about why this is important to you.

This example shows how a few well-chosen words can drive the conversation toward change talk. Had the practitioner only used the reflection, it most likely would have gone more like this:

> CLIENT: Thinking about what and when to eat is a constant stress and some days I'm just too tired. [sustain talk]
>
> PRACTITIONER: You've been through a lot, and some days it wears you down. [reflection]
>
> CLIENT: I just don't know what to do anymore. [sustain talk]

Reflections are powerful tools that encourage clients to expand on a subject. People will tend to give you more of what you've reflected. In this case, the reflection only validated the client's feelings of hopelessness, ultimately encouraging more sustain talk. By adding the affirmation to the reflection, you are able to validate his feeling and reframe it into a positive and motivating statement.

Affirmations Decrease Defensiveness

While the ultimate goal of affirmations is to set the stage for change talk, they can also be used to help mollify defensiveness. For example, a client is referred by his doctor to a dietetics practitioner for nutrition education after being told his cholesterol is too high. The client is visibly agitated as the appointment begins, with his arms crossed against his abdomen and looks at the practitioner with a cold expression.

> CLIENT: I don't even know what I'm supposed to be doing here.
>
> PRACTITIONER: You're unsure about your purpose here today. [reflection]

CLIENT: No, I know I have to get my cholesterol down. I don't know what *you're* going to do about it.

PRACTITIONER: You're used to doing things on your own. [affirmation]

CLIENT: Well if I don't, no one else will.

PRACTITIONER: You're right, it is completely up to you. [reflection that supports autonomy] I can help if you'd like my help. [ask permission] What's the best use of our time together today? [open-ended question]

The affirmation, reflection, and open-ended question voiced by the practitioner supported client autonomy. Instead of arguing for why she could help him, the practitioner reframed the client's statement, "I know I have to get my cholesterol down. I don't know what you're going to do about it," into an affirmation. It's not uncommon for people to enter counseling sessions with apprehension and defensiveness, especially if it wasn't their idea to come in the first place. Engaging the client and understanding his perspective is an important part of dismantling his defensiveness.

CRAFTING AFFIRMATIONS

Affirmations are a type of complex reflection. Similar to a "continue the paragraph" reflection described in more detail in Chapter 8, the practitioner must interpret what the client has said and make a guess about what kind of positive efforts the client has demonstrated. In order to avoid making the client feel judged, focus an affirmation around specific behaviors or characteristics instead of attitudes, decisions, or goals.

"Running that 5K showed you that you're capable of far more than you previously thought."
"Talking to your mom about how she nitpicks about your food choices took an incredible amount of courage."

Play it safe when crafting affirmations. Pick a characteristic you are certain the person possesses. If the client disagrees with you and begins to focus on why she does not agree with the statement, the whole focus of the appointment can be sidetracked.

When crafting affirmations avoid starting with "I." You are not the focus, the client is.

Although affirmations are positive statements regarding one's character or values, they are not the same as giving praise or compliments. There is a difference between giving compliments and strategically using affirmations. A compliment has a tone of judgment or evaluation made by the practitioner. When crafting affirmations avoid starting with "I." You are not the focus, the client is. Here are some examples of compliments and affirmations:

Compliment: "You look great!"

versus

Affirmation: "You worked hard this week and made it to all your workouts."

Praise: "I'm so proud of you!"

versus

Affirmation: "You feel really good about what you've accomplished."

Compliments and praise are not bad; they do give positive reinforcement to specific behaviors. The downside emerges when clients get into the habit of making changes for their practitioner's approval instead of for their intrinsic value. You might be thinking, "But change is good no matter what, right?" The potential problem has to do with what happens when the client stops doing well. Using the example above, if next week the client doesn't feel like he looks great, he may be too ashamed or embarrassed to come back.

It is important to note that in order for an affirmation to be believable, it must be genuine. Some people are more likely to internalize insults and put-downs, so affirmations may be responded to with denial, ignorance, or total dismissal. This may be the case if an affirmation is given with a tone of superiority or mockery. As the practitioner, your tone of voice and facial expression will tell the client whether you are sincere. Notice the effect your affirmations have on the client. Some cultures do not respond well to them. Read your clients and let them guide you.

Make it your goal to hunt for authentic examples of positive characteristics within the client's commentary. It all starts when you pick up the scent in a seemingly insignificant client statement. Ask open-ended questions to have the client elaborate more. Follow the trail of information until you find a strength you can acknowledge. Then present the affirmation as a statement: "It's through your cooking that you are showing your family how much you love them. You are a caring person." Below are some brief scripts in which the practitioner seeks opportunities to use affirmations.

Here is an example of a 70-year old woman who struggles with mild depression and motivation to exercise:

CLIENT: I was just so much better at this when I did it before.

PRACTITIONER: Tell me about that time. [open-ended question]

CLIENT: I could get up in the morning and exercise first thing.

PRACTITIONER: You were able to make exercise a top priority. [reflection]

CLIENT: Well, I just knew it would make me feel better, and it really did. My therapist used to beg me to exercise. I felt like it worked better than my meds. I even slept better.

PRACTITIONER: Exercising keeps your energy levels up and helps to subdue the depression, keeping you in a healthier place. [reflection]

CLIENT: I think that I can get up in the morning and walk around the outdoor mall near my house. It's not that big of a deal. I just need to think about how good it's going to make me feel.

PRACTITIONER: You're committed to making this a priority because you know how much you'll benefit from it. [affirmation]

CLIENT: Yes, it really points my whole day in a different direction. I know it sounds small, but I just do so much better when I start the day on the right foot.

In this dialogue, the client mentions how she was able to exercise in the past. Halfway through the dialogue, the practitioner switches the reflection into the present tense, implying that the benefits the client felt would be the same if she started exercising again. The client was then able to visualize herself getting up in the morning to go for a walk and she decided it was possible.

In the next example, a 45-year-old woman is trying to plan and prepare regularly scheduled meals for herself.

PRACTITIONER: How is your meal schedule going? [open-ended question]

CLIENT: It's going OK. I've been making an effort to have my lunch in the break room at work instead of at my desk. That way I don't work and eat at the same time.

PRACTITIONER: You made a point of getting away from your desk so you'll be more focused on eating. [reflection]

CLIENT: Yes, because if I sit at my desk and eat, before you know it my lunch is gone and I didn't really taste any of it.

PRACTITIONER: And it's important to you to be more mindful of how your body feels when you're eating so you feel more satisfied. [reflection]

CLIENT: It has been lately, at least. I can see that I've been eating so much and hardly tasting any of it. It's like I've been eating in a fog.

PRACTITIONER: You want to do what's right for your body. [affirmation]

CLIENT: I really do. It just feels right.

Accepting	Committed	Flexible	Persevering	Stubborn
Active	Competent	Focused	Persistent	Thankful
Adaptable	Concerned	Forgiving	Positive	Thorough
Adventuresome	Confident	Forward-looking	Powerful	Thoughtful
Affectionate	Considerate	Free	Prayerful	Tough
Affirmative	Courageous	Happy	Quick	Trusting
Alert	Creative	Healthy	Reasonable	Trustworthy
Alive	Decisive	Hopeful	Receptive	Truthful
Ambitious	Dedicated	Imaginative	Relaxed	Understanding
Anchored	Determined	Ingenious	Reliable	Unique
Assertive	Die-hard	Intelligent	Resourceful	Unstoppable
Assured	Diligent	Knowledgeable	Responsible	Vigorous
Attentive	Doer	Loving	Sensible	Visionary
Bold	Eager	Mature	Skillful	Whole
Brave	Earnest	Open	Solid	Willing
Bright	Effective	Optimistic	Spiritual	Winning
Capable	Energetic	Orderly	Stable	Wise
Careful	Experienced	Organized	Steady	Worthy
Cheerful	Faithful	Patient	Straight	Zealous
Clever	Fearless	Perceptive	Strong	Zestful

FIGURE 7.2. Characteristics of successful changers. From Miller (2004).

PICKING THE RIGHT AFFIRMATION

There are many ways to offer affirmations depending on which direction you'd like to guide your client. Figure 7.2 offers a list of 100 characteristics of successful people. It can be used to help give you an idea of what you're looking for in your clients.

Below are two scenarios, each with a list of affirming words that might be appropriate to the situation.

Scenario 1

Tyler is a 55-year-old electrician who has just been diagnosed with celiac disease, a condition requiring a strict gluten-free diet. He has spent his entire life eating wheat, barley, and rye, the three main food sources of gluten. He is now being asked to restrict gluten entirely. He has returned for his first follow-up appointment and has eliminated gluten for an entire week. It wasn't easy, but he feels successful. The following characteristics may be appropriate for Tyler.

Adaptable	Effective
Capable	Flexible
Committed	Focused

Competent	Imaginative
Confident	Knowledgeable
Creative	Persistent
Dedicated	Resourceful
Determined	Thorough
Diligent	Tough

It's easy to affirm clients when they are successful. It's harder to do so when they are struggling. Consider affirmations that might be used with the client in Scenario 2.

Scenario 2

Becky is a 45-year-old mother of three who has end-stage renal failure after a traumatic car accident damaged her only functioning kidney. She has just started dialysis and needs to restrict her intake of fluids, potassium, phosphorus, and sodium. She also needs to increase her protein intake, a nutrient she previously had to limit. Possible affirmations for Becky include the following:

Brave	Courageous
Capable	Hopeful
Careful	Organized
Committed	Persevering
Competent	Strong
Concerned	Tough

Which affirmation the practitioner chooses depends on what he or she wants the client to talk about more. When affirming a client, there is no right or wrong answer. There are many ways to affirm clients, and any affirmation is better than no affirmation. Each affirmation will take the client on a specific path. As mentioned before, you are likely to get more of what you affirm or reflect. If you reflect sustain talk, the client is certain to dwell on how her previous attempt failed. If you highlight the client's strengths or commitment, then you are likely going to hear more change talk.

Test Yourself

Below are client statements followed by three possible affirmations. As you read the client statement, think of possible qualities to affirm before looking at the three affirmations provided.

- *Client statement*: "It's not that I don't want to eat healthy. I've done it before. I used to go to the store and get all the right foods, but then they started going bad in the fridge and I couldn't stand all that waste."

- *Affirmation 1*: "You want to eat healthy."
- *Affirmation 2*: "You already know what kind of foods to buy."
- *Affirmation 3*: "Not being wasteful is important to you."

- *Client statement*: "I just felt so much better when I was working out in my garden. It's not even that I was exercising all that hard. I was just always doing something."
- *Affirmation 1*: "You have a green thumb."
- *Affirmation 2*: "It's not about exercise to you, it's about cultivating something."
- *Affirmation 3*: "You notice that it's easy for you to incorporate physical activity when you do the things you enjoy."

- *Client statement*: "That's why gastric bypass is right for me. I can do it. I know I can, I just need help. These past few months have shown me what I'm capable of. I've never eaten better in my life, but the weight just won't budge."
- *Affirmation 1*: "You are committed to getting your body as healthy as possible before this surgery."
- *Affirmation 2*: "You have proven to yourself how strong you are."
- *Affirmation 3*: "You are capable of amazing things. Nothing is going to stand in your way."

- *Client statement*: "It's hard to see how much strength I've lost over the years. I can still do most things though; I just don't recover the way I used to. Every year, I take my girls and their families on a ski trip. Lately, I see myself starting to slow down. You know, though, it's not a race. I just enjoy being out there on that mountain with my whole family and I feel good."
- *Affirmation 1*: "You enjoy being active with your family."
- *Affirmation 2*: "Being there for your family is important to you and you're able to shift your focus to what's important."
- *Affirmation 3*: "You just cruise down the mountain enjoying the big picture. You feel peace in where you are in your life."

- *Client statement*: "My biggest problem is soda. I drink about two a day now and I think I'm addicted to it. I was drinking more than that and I cut it back already. I just need that caffeine in the afternoon to stay alert at work."
- *Affirmation 1*: "You were already successful with making a change in how much soda you drink."

- *Affirmation 2*: "You know yourself well and where you'd like to focus your attention."
- *Affirmation 3*: "Your career is important to you and you want to finish strong each day."

SELF-AFFIRMATIONS

Although affirmations help clients to internalize and develop positive self-talk, the best type of affirmation is the one the client generates. The use of strengths-based open-ended questions can help you to uncover self-affirmations that become even more powerful in the behavior change process.

> PRACTITIONER: Tell me about some things you do to take care of your son's health. [strengths-based question]
>
> CLIENT: I do always make a point of putting together his lunch. I just worry that he'll be tired in his afternoon classes if he doesn't have a healthy lunch.
>
> PRACTITIONER: You're looking out for him. [reflection]
>
> CLIENT: I just love him and want him to have a long, healthy life. [self-affirmation]

In this example the practitioner asks the client to come up with something she does for her son's health. By asking the client to come up with positive behaviors, the client is more likely to internalize it, letting it spread to other areas of her life.

Sometimes affirmations made by the practitioner produce a domino effect resulting in a client self-affirmation. Here is an example of a 65-year-old woman who had an elevated fasting glucose lab.

> CLIENT: All my sisters have diabetes and my mother too.
>
> PRACTITIONER: And it worries you that you're next. [reflection]
>
> CLIENT: Yes, I'm scared that if I don't change what I'm doing now, that I'm going to get it too.
>
> PRACTITIONER: You see that there are some things you can do that might reduce your chances of developing diabetes. [reflection]
>
> CLIENT: I do. I think I need to quit drinking soda, for one. I go through a 12-pack a week. I think that's where I need to start.
>
> PRACTITIONER: Once you see your goal, you don't back down. [affirmation]
>
> CLIENT: Yes, I'm a goal-driven person. I've always been that way. [self-affirmation]

PRACTITIONER: What's another time that you made a goal and went for it? [open-ended question]

In the previous dialogue, the client starts to voice change talk. The practitioner follows with an affirmation to help solidify her commitment. The client then makes a powerful strengths-based statement about herself. The practitioner can strategically use that statement as a springboard to elicit more positive statements. It can also be used in future dialogues to help further cement her commitment to change.

There's never a bad time or place for an affirmation. Always be on the lookout for a characteristic or attribute to affirm. Including affirmations in the mix with open-ended questions, reflections and summaries will increase your client's confidence in behavior change.

CHAPTER 8

Reflections

I don't know what it is about listening. I just know when I'm heard, it feels damned good.
—CARL ROGERS

It feels good to be validated. Clients feel heard and understood when the practitioner takes the time to reflect or paraphrase what they are saying. With reflective listening, the most widely used microskill in MI, the practitioner reflects what the client is thinking and feeling and expresses this understanding back to the client. A general guideline is to provide two reflections or more for every open-ended question. Reflective listening statements do more than just demonstrate that the practitioner is listening; they are intentionally and strategically placed to emphasize the client's ambivalence, strengths, and desire to change. This chapter introduces this important microskill within MI that becomes the foundation for an environment where clients can feel supported in their efforts toward change.

BENEFITS OF REFLECTIONS

Consistent and liberal use of reflections makes the client feel validated and understood, ultimately building trust within the counseling relationship.

Consistent and liberal use of reflections makes the client feel validated and understood, which ultimately builds trust within the counseling relationship.

Rephrasing what the client says demonstrates empathy and a general curiosity and desire to fully understand the client's perspective. Reflections also help to coax the client to elaborate on certain thoughts and feelings. In hearing his own thoughts and feelings laid out in a direct and organized way, the client may even experience an "ah-ha" moment. A client might say, "Gosh, I never realized I felt that way."

FORMING REFLECTIONS

In reflective listening, also known as active listening, the practitioner interprets what the person means and relays this meaning back to the client. Reflections are statements, not questions; therefore voice inflection decreases at the end of the statement. Reflections open with statements such as:

"So you feel. . . . "
"You're wondering if. . . . "
"It seems as though. . . . "
"You are. . . . "

Reflections are concise. In general, attempt to make the reflection no longer than the client's original statement. Forming accurate reflections requires you to listen intently not only to what the person says, but also to what the person means to say. People don't always say what they mean, so at times, you will be taking a guess at what you think they mean.

CLIENT: This just came out of nowhere. I don't have diabetes.

PRACTITIONER: You don't see yourself as a person who can have this kind of disease.

CLIENT: I've been through Vietnam.

PRACTITIONER: You thought that your fighting was over.

Tone of voice is the difference between expressing empathy or sarcasm. If you genuinely place yourself in a curious frame of mind, you may find your voice naturally adopts an empathetic cadence. Strive to be a clear pool of water, reflecting the image of what people intend to be.

Strive to be a clear pool of water, reflecting the image of what people intend to be.

WHEN TO REFLECT

A general rule of thumb is to reflect after almost every client statement. However, there are three especially important times to reflect what you hear.

Reflect When You Hear Change Talk

This is the heart of MI. Clients often express reasons to make a behavior change, a need to change, plans for change, or even a previous occasion they were successful at changing. In reflecting change talk, clients hear their own positive feelings about change, ultimately fueling that desire.

> CLIENT: I know I could save a lot of money if I ate out less often, but that means I'd have to cook more. It's not that I can't cook. I'm actually a really good cook. I think I'm just being lazy.
>
> PRACTITIONER: You recognize a few benefits of making your own meals at home more often and even believe you have the skills to do so. [reflects change talk]

Reflect When You Hear the Client Express Ambivalence

Clients may not be aware of their mixed feelings about the behavior change. By hearing both sides of the argument restated, they may start to understand why they haven't already made the behavior change on their own. It's also another opportunity to hear again reasons in favor of changing.

> CLIENT: I really want to train for this 10K my friend is doing. It would be so good for me. But I just don't have the time.
>
> PRACTITIONER: You're not sure how to fit the training into your schedule and the thought of training for an event like this excites you. [double-sided reflection]

Reflect When You Hear the Client Express Sustain Talk

In reflecting the client's hesitation, you can test the waters to assess motivation and increase the client's awareness of current concerns regarding the behavior change. Reflecting sustain talk isn't *always* the best tactic; too much emphasis on sustain talk can leave your client feeling stuck and hopeless. However, on occasion, reflecting sustain talk may be very powerful.

> CLIENT: I don't think my diet is that bad.
>
> PRACTITIONER: You're not sure you need to make any changes to your diet. [amplified reflection]

In reflecting change talk, clients hear their own positive feelings about change, ultimately fueling that desire.

While simply reflecting sustain talk will make the client feel understood, reframing the sustain talk or using an amplified reflection can help nudge the client through ambivalence. What you emphasize in your reflections depends on your client and his or her readiness to change.

CLIENT: I don't think my diet is that bad.

PRACTITIONER: There are some aspects of your diet that are quite healthy. [reframe] Tell me about those.

TYPES OF REFLECTIONS

Reflections are often categorized into two groups: simple and complex. Simple reflections repeat or slightly rephrase elements of the client's statement. Complex reflections add further or alternative meaning beyond what the client has just said.

Simple versus Complex Reflections

Simple reflections are especially useful at the beginning of an appointment while building rapport. Notice the simple reflections in the following initial interaction:

PRACTITIONER: Mia, tell me about yourself.

CLIENT: I work part-time as a teacher's aide at my son's school. I have three children; two are in high school and then my son is in the fourth grade. I've never seen a nutritionist before, so I don't really know what to expect today.

PRACTITIONER: Today is your first appointment with a nutritionist and you're wondering what to expect.

CLIENT: Yeah, I'm not really sure how this works, but I saw your advertisement at the library and there was something that really resonated with me on your flier.

PRACTITIONER: It was a flier at the library that brought you in today. What about the flier spoke to you?

CLIENT: I liked how you said that you could help people heal their relationship with food. I never thought of food as a relationship, but I guess just like anything else, it's more complex than I had realized.

PRACTITIONER: You'd like to explore your relationship with food today because there's something there that seems complicated.

While simple reflections are helpful in the beginning of an appointment, overuse can result in the client feeling parroted and sends conversations into circles. Complex reflections, especially those that emphasize change talk, move the client forward, enhancing motivation for change. Often, in order to say what's not yet been spoken, the practitioner must make a guess at the meaning behind the client's statement.

A complex reflection may emphasize feelings or the emotional dimension of what the client has said. Consider the two different practitioner responses to the following client statement. The simple reflection repeats back what the client said, whereas the complex reflection moves the client forward into exploring the origins of her negative body image:

- *Client statement*: "Growing up, my mom always complained about her weight. She was always dieting and making us eat her diet food."
- *Simple reflection*: "Growing up, you had to eat your mom's diet food."
- *Complex reflection*: "Your mom put everyone on her diet, making you feel deprived at times and wondering if your body wasn't OK either."

There are many ways to provide complex reflections. A certain type of reflection may fit the occasion depending on what you know about the client and the client's readiness to change. Sometimes it might be helpful to understate the reflection, whereas at other times it might help to overstate or even amplify the reflection, gently guiding the client to consider other angles. Sometimes just the right metaphor can be used to drive home an emotion.

Metaphors

A metaphor, simile, or analogy can help bring a concept to life. Comparing what the client says to an object or action helps emphasize the complexity of the client's feelings. Often words can be rather limiting. By using a metaphor the practitioner paints a picture of how the client may feel. The imagery provides a new way to look at what was said, ultimately deepening the client's understanding.

CLIENT: I feel all over the place. One minute I'm counting calories, trying to be "good" with my eating, and the next minute I'm throwing in the towel and bingeing on a pan of brownies.

PRACTITIONER: Dieting can feel like a rollercoaster ride. Before you know it, you're upside down.

Reframing

A reframe is simply a reflection that highlights a different perspective within the client's statement. It's particularly useful to deemphasize sustain talk. A practitioner may hear sustain talk and recast the statement into a neutral statement, change talk, or an affirmation. Here are some examples:

CLIENT: I feel bad going to the gym after work because I hardly see my kids as it is.

PRACTITIONER: It's important to you to be there for your kids.

CLIENT: I'm just here because my doctor told me to come.

PRACTITIONER: You trust your doctor and you're wondering how I might be able to help.

CLIENT: I tried eating my dinner at the table without the TV on, like you had suggested, and I got more anxious and even lonely.

PRACTITIONER: While it didn't turn out how you were hoping, you were mindful of your thoughts and feelings during this experiment.

CLIENT: I notice that I don't feel good after I eat a lot of junk food.

PRACTITIONER: You know your body well.

Reframing the client's seemingly negative statements into neutral or even positive reflections will likely affirm the client and direct her forward instead of allowing her to dwell on the negative aspects of behavior change.

Continuing the Paragraph

Reflections that continue the paragraph take a guess at what is unstated but implied in the conversation. These reflections move the client forward, sometimes moving the conversation in a new direction. Continuing the paragraph is not the same as finishing someone's sentence. Finishing someone's sentence is discouraged in counseling, because it can interrupt the client's train of thought. However, continuing the paragraph can help bring up new pieces of the puzzle in exploring ambivalence about a change.

CLIENT: I'd like to go on walks with my sister. She's a perfect workout buddy because she goes my pace. Her life is so hectic though.

PRACTITIONER: And you're concerned she may not be reliable.

In addition, continuing the paragraph reflections can take what the client says and accentuate any spoken or unspoken change talk.

CLIENT: I'm tired of being tired. I drink way too many energy drinks.

PRACTITIONER: And you want to make a change that naturally boosts your energy levels.

There is often crossover between the different types of reflections. For example, continuing the paragraph can also reframe the client's original statement, reflecting on what the client said from a new angle.

CLIENT: I hate my thighs and bottom. I feel like people are always looking at those areas of my body.

PRACTITIONER: And there are other things about you you'd like them to notice.

Double-Sided

Double-sided reflections are used when the client is expressing ambivalence. When the client is sharing both advantages and disadvantages of making a behavior change, it can be productive to reflect back the expressed ambivalence so the client better understands his conflicted feelings. Double-sided reflections often start with "On one hand . . . ," and finish with "On the other hand. . . . " When providing a double-sided reflection, connect both sides with "and" instead of "but" in order to give both choices equal weight.

CLIENT: I know I need to switch to diet sodas, but I just can't stand the taste of fake sugar.

PRACTITIONER: On one hand you're not so sure about the taste of artificial sweeteners and on the other hand, you are concerned about how regular soda may affect your blood sugars.

By reflecting the ambivalence you guide the client to consider the importance of both sides. However, at times the client will get stuck in his ambivalence, at which time it is best to use reflections that only emphasize the change talk.

Reflecting both the change talk and sustain talk demonstrates empathy for the challenge of making a change. When using double-sided reflections, start by reflecting the sustain talk and end with the change talk. This strategy will increase the chance that the client responds with more change talk.

Consider the two double-sided reflections below and the order of sustain talk and change talk:

CLIENT: I've thought about riding my bike to work, [change talk] but I'm afraid I'm going to be a sweaty mess when I get there. [sustain talk]

PRACTITIONER: You'd like to somehow work exercise into your commute [change talk] and you're concerned that doing so would make you feel sweaty all day. [sustain talk]

CLIENT: Yes, I'm afraid of how I would look and I'd just feel dirty the rest of the day. [sustain talk]

CLIENT: I've thought about riding my bike to work, [change talk] but I'm afraid I'm going to be a sweaty mess when I get there. [sustain talk]

PRACTITIONER: Sweating is a concern, [sustain talk] and somehow working exercise into your commute remains appealing. [change talk]

CLIENT: Yes, I'm jealous of the people I see ride past me on bikes when I'm stuck in traffic. [change talk]

When the practitioner ended with change talk, the client spoke more change talk. When the practitioner ended with sustain talk, the client spoke more sustain talk. While this isn't always the case, clients are more likely to respond to the end of the practitioner's statement. Therefore, by reflecting the change talk last, you may propel your client forward toward change.

Undershooting

An undershooting reflection might be used at times to encourage continued exploration. The undershooting reflection depreciates the intensity of the emotion expressed. Doing so may encourage the client to clarify what was meant which can deepen the client's understanding of her feelings.

CLIENT: I hate that my husband eats whatever he wants in front of me. He knows I'm trying to watch what I eat and it makes it so much harder for me to watch him eating things I can't have.

PRACTITIONER: You're not crazy about your husband's eating habits.

CLIENT: More than that, it makes me crazy and a little resentful.

Undershooting reflections can bring out the client's true emotion. They are especially useful when clients aren't sure they should feel a certain way.

Amplified

An amplified reflection involves reflecting back what the person has said in an exaggerated form. This technique may encourage the client to back off a bit or consider another side of personal ambivalence. It's important to provide amplified reflections in an empathetic manner, free of sarcasm.

CLIENT: I'm just so busy. I don't know how other people do it. I go to work and when I come home I'm exhausted. When am I supposed to work out?

PRACTITIONER: There is just no space in your day for physical activity.

CLIENT: Well, I don't know. Maybe. I know a few guys get together right after work and go to the gym. If I was going to work out, it would have to be then because once I'm home I'm not leaving again.

Understated and amplified reflections are used sparingly, as regularly overstating or understating client statements can result in clients not feeling heard or understood. It's best to err on the side of undershooting, since it seems to help clients continue exploring their emotions. Figure 8.1 provides a summary of the different types of reflections along with additional examples.

REFLECTING STRATEGICALLY

A skilled practitioner knows when to use each type of reflection. In general, simple reflections are best when you're first getting to know a client. Once you've built rapport, complex reflections are best for moving forward and unpacking deeper meaning. Novices will often say, "I feel like I'm just being annoying when I constantly repeat what the client is saying." In general, echoing what the client is saying will get old after a while. If you feel like a broken record and you're just going around in circles with the client, you're relying too heavily on simple reflections.

Simple reflections are typically neutral and stabilizing; although they help build rapport, they don't often result in change talk within the appointment. One way to move the conversation toward change talk is to use complex reflections instead of simple, stabilizing reflections. Reframing, double-sided, or continuing the paragraph are forward-moving complex reflections that help emphasize change talk. With any one of these, the practitioner is guessing at what is unsaid but implied. Consider the following stabilizing versus forward-moving reflections:

- *Client statement*: "I know I'm supposed to eat vegetables, but I'm just not a big fan of them."
- *Stabilizing reflection*: "You don't care much for vegetables."
- *Forward-moving reflection*: "You're not crazy about vegetables and yet you know they have certain health benefits, so you're wondering how you might be able to incorporate them in a pleasant way."

Type of reflection	Definition	Example
Simple	Contains little or no additional content beyond what the client has said.	"You walked for an hour yesterday."
Complex	Adds more or different meaning beyond what the client has just said; a guess as to what the client may have meant.	"The pressure of the gym membership adds a layer of guilt you don't like and you prefer being outside in the open air."
Metaphor	A word or phrase denoting one object or action used in place of another, suggesting likeness or analogy between them.	"The appointment with your doctor lit a fire within and got you thinking about being active again."
Reframing	Places the client's statement in a new light, giving new perspective.	"You like the idea of being in nature and getting some fresh air."
Continuing the paragraph	The practitioner offers what might be the next (as yet unspoken) sentence in the client's paragraph.	"You're more motivated to exercise when you can be outside."
Double-sided	Includes both client *sustain talk* and *change talk*, usually with the conjunction "and."	"On the one hand, you don't like working out at the gym, and on the other hand, you're feeling more motivated to be active since meeting with your doctor."
Undershooting	Diminishes or understates the intensity of the content or emotion expressed by a client	"Some days the gym doesn't do it for you."
Amplified	Reflects back the client's content with greater intensity than the client had expressed; one form of response to client *sustain talk* or *discord*.	"You hate exercising indoors."

FIGURE 8.1. Types of reflections. For each type of reflection there is a reflective listening response to the following client statement: "Gym memberships haven't worked well for me in the past. I never end up going and then I always feel guilty about the money I wasted. I haven't done much the last few months, but after my appointment with the doctor yesterday, I came home and went for an hour-long walk."

- *Client statement*: "I don't know how we're supposed to eat better. My husband wastes all our money on his stupid cigarettes and online poker games. It doesn't leave us much to work with each month. I don't know what to do."
- *Stabilizing reflection*: "You feel stuck."
- *Forward-moving reflection*: "You want to provide your family with balanced meals and if you just knew what to do, you would do it."

- *Client statement*: "I probably sound like the worst mother. I know I'm not supposed to give my 2-year-old so much juice, but she runs around the house yelling, "Duce, duce, duce!" and it's so cute. Plus, she throws a big fit when I just give her water."
- *Stabilizing reflection*: "It's hard to say no to your toddler."
- *Forward-moving reflection*: "You feel torn. It's hard to say no to your toddler and at the same time you want what's best for her."

In each scenario above, you'll notice that the stabilizing reflection is not necessarily "wrong" and may even be a better choice at times. The forward-moving reflections simply provide more momentum to affirm the client, take a guess at change talk, or encourage the client to consider other pieces of the puzzle.

There's really no such thing as a wrong reflection. Some reflections help the client move forward more than others, but you can never go wrong by providing a reflection. No matter what kind, as long as the tone is appropriate, you will always demonstrate empathy and a desire to understand the client. And if your reflection doesn't quite represent what the client meant, he or she will correct you and still appreciate your efforts toward listening and understanding.

> There's really no such thing as a wrong reflection.

If reflective listening is new to you, begin by being consistent with reflecting after most client statements. Once you become used to the consistency of reflections, then you may find it easier to attend to the types of reflections that can best help move the client forward. Don't overthink reflections. It's asking a lot for a practitioner to think of the best type of reflection and then how to say it all in a split second. Instead of focusing on the type of reflection you want to provide, think instead about the change talk and how to best express that piece back to the client. Different types of reflections will naturally flow with practice.

The script below includes a variety of reflections. Notice the progression from simple reflections to more complex reflections that include forward-moving language.

PRACTITIONER: Hi, James. Do you go by "James?"

CLIENT: Yes, you can call me that, but most people call me Jimmy.

PRACTITIONER: Great, then if it's OK with you, I'll call you Jimmy too.

CLIENT: That's fine.

PRACTITIONER: Jimmy, your doctor sent you to me today because I'm a health coach and there were some behaviors she was concerned about. I have here that you are 15 years old and in high school. Is there anything else I should know about you?

CLIENT: I don't know. That's probably all you need to know. My doctor told me she doesn't want me drinking so much soda and playing so many video games.

PRACTITIONER: Right, video games and soda—that's what she wrote here too. [simple reflection] What are your thoughts on being here today?

CLIENT: I'm not crazy about it, but I know I'm not the healthiest.

PRACTITIONER: You see yourself as not all that healthy. [simple reflection] Tell me more about that.

CLIENT: I don't eat that great and then there's this "pudge." I have this reputation at school as being the kid who eats anything and everything. I've even had friends challenge me to eating contests.

PRACTITIONER: Because of your larger size, kids have you pegged as someone with a certain eating style. [simple reflection] What's that like?

CLIENT: I mean it's cool. I guess I get attention or whatever, but it's also kind of stupid because any time I do an eating contest with someone I feel sick afterward.

PRACTITIONER: On one hand you like the attention from your friends, and on the other hand you'd like to be known for other cool things you can do because the eating thing is getting old. [double-sided and continuing the paragraph reflections]

CLIENT: Yeah.

PRACTITIONER: What are the other cool things that you do?

CLIENT: I don't know. I guess I'm good at math. And video games. I can beat anyone in Combat Commando.

PRACTITIONER: All right, a gift for numbers. That's cool! [affirmation] And, that's right—you're good at video games. Between the two things your doctor mentioned, video games and sodas, which, if any, interest you today to talk about?

CLIENT: Well, if I'm going to give up the eating contests, then I'm still going to need to beat my friends at video games. So probably the soda.

PRACTITIONER: That makes sense; I'm sure the video gaming requires regular practice, so let's leave that one alone for now. How do you feel about the soda?

CLIENT: Well, obviously I like it. It helps me stay awake so I can play more video games.

PRACTITIONER: You like the taste and the caffeine buzz. [simple reflection]

CLIENT: Yeah.

PRACTITIONER: You really like soda, and yet you chose cutting that back as a change you'd be up for trying out. [double-sided reflection] What are some reasons to make this change right now?

CLIENT: I totally didn't realize I drank that many until my mom pointed it out to the doctor. When I heard her say I went through a six-pack of Mountain Dew in a day, I was like, dude, that's pretty bad.

PRACTITIONER: So it sounds like a lot to you. [simple reflection] What else? What are some other reasons to make this change?

CLIENT: Well, there's the "pudge." I'm sure there are calories or whatever in those drinks. I'm sure the extra around my middle can't be good for me.

PRACTITIONER: You're wondering about the association between weight and health and you're thinking that drinking fewer cans of soda might result in losing a few pounds. [continuing the paragraph reflection]

CLIENT: Yeah, plus I gotta get a date to prom someday.

PRACTITIONER: You're afraid some girls at school might judge a book by its cover. [metaphor reflection] What concerns you most about your current soda habit?

CLIENT: I have an older cousin who's in his 30s and he's built like me. He actually got me started on Mountain Dew. He just got diabetes. I don't really know what that is, but I know he has to prick himself all the time and I hate needles.

PRACTITIONER: Needles totally freak you out. [amplified reflection]

CLIENT: Yeah, I don't know how he does it.

PRACTITIONER: You'd like to cut back on soda because you don't want diabetes and watching your cousin go through all of that has you worried. You've also shared that you don't want to be someone who drinks a six-pack a day and even wonder if cutting back might change your appearance. [summary]

CLIENT: Yeah, now my cousin has to eat all healthy and stuff. We'll see how long he lasts on his rabbit food. My aunt said he'll probably stick with it for a few months and then go back to the soda and junk.

PRACTITIONER: It sounds like your family isn't very optimistic that your cousin can sustain the change. [complex reflection] What do you think?

CLIENT: I don't know; it can't be that hard.

PRACTITIONER: You'd like to see him stick it out because he's someone you look up to. [continuing the paragraph reflection]

CLIENT: Yeah, I guess.

PRACTITIONER: What do you think your cousin would say about you cutting back on soda?

CLIENT: He'd tell me to do it.

PRACTITIONER: You have his support. [simple reflection] Who else might support you in this change?

CLIENT: My mom. She'll probably nag me to death.

PRACTITIONER: So she'll be cheering you on, but possibly not in the way you'd like her to. [complex reflection]

CLIENT: Yeah.

PRACTITIONER: How do you want her to help?

CLIENT: She could probably stop buying so much of it at the store. But she drinks it too, and so does my older sister.

PRACTITIONER: So maybe she could help you by letting you make this change on your own and not nagging you, but also helping out by making it a little harder to get the sodas. You probably want other people in the house cutting back on soda too. [continuing the paragraph reflection]

CLIENT: Yeah, they can do whatever they want, but it would make it easier if everyone was allowed a certain number of sodas each week and like we all had our own stash.

PRACTITIONER: You have an idea for how this could work. [affirmation] Tell me more about how you might make this change, if you were to make it.

Reflections are a useful way of communicating with others, both in your work with patients, and in your personal relationships. Make a conscious effort to understand others and communicate that understanding through reflective listening. Relationships that had once been foggy under a blanket of misunderstanding can miraculously become as clear as a morning after a rainstorm. People feel connected to one another through understanding, compassion, and support, all of which are communicated through the strategic use of reflections.

CHAPTER 9

Summaries

> Listen carefully for the heart and essence of what the client
> has said, succinctly stringing together pearls that capture
> strength, resiliency, effort, aspirations, confidence, and
> motivations for change, adorning the client with a pearl
> necklace summary of change talk.
> —STEVEN M. BERG-SMITH

Reflective listening goes beyond just the short reflections highlighting client statements. Reflections emphasizing ambivalence and change talk are linked together to create summaries giving the client a bird's-eye view of his own thoughts and feelings about a behavior. When these summaries are sprinkled throughout the appointment, the client–practitioner rapport is enhanced, as the client continues to feel heard, supported, and understood.

A reflection is like a small mirror that the practitioner holds up for the client to see experiences and feelings that are spoken. A hand-held mirror provides only a limited view. If a reflection is a hand-held mirror, then a full-length mirror would be a summary. The summary provides the client with a full view of key pieces that have been shared. The client has the opportunity to step back and see the entire view from a new vantage point.

This chapter provides an overview of the benefits of summaries and strategies for providing meaningful summaries. Combined with open-ended question (O), affirmations (A), and reflections (R), summaries (S) are the final instrument in the OARS orchestra. Together, the OARS create a rhythm within a counseling session that is demonstrated through a full appointment script at the end of the chapter.

BENEFITS OF SUMMARIES

Summaries provide another opportunity for the client to hear ambivalent thoughts or a genuine desire to change. Just like reflections, summaries provide evidence that the practitioner is listening. Through grouping several key rephrased statements together, the practitioner can help the client to organize or make sense of thoughts and feelings. A reflection is like a single small pearl offered to the client that represents a meaningful shared insight. A practitioner simply strings the pearls together every now and then and presents the complete strand back to the client.

Summaries can be especially useful in transitioning the conversation from one topic to another or to draw a client back from an off-topic tangent. Summaries are like roundabout traffic circles that help improve the flow of traffic and easily allow for a direction change or continued forward movement. When a driver approaches a traffic circle, he or she circles around and can continue straight in the same direction or head in a new direction. Similarly, summaries allow the conversation to circle around the topic and then either continue discussing the same topic or allow for a smooth transition in a new direction.

> *Summaries are like roundabout traffic circles that help improve the flow of traffic and easily allow for a direction change or continued forward movement.*

TIPS FOR PROVIDING MEANINGFUL SUMMARIES

When providing a summary, there's no need to revisit every point the client makes. Only revisit the essential thoughts or feelings that will move the client forward toward contemplating or committing to behavior change. Choose summary components strategically as if you are selecting flowers to create a beautiful bouquet for the client. If you were making a bouquet, you wouldn't include every flower in the field. You would consider the different colors, styles, and condition of the petals. You would only select those that are beautiful and complementary to each other.

> *When providing a summary, there's no need to revisit every point the client makes. Only revisit the essential thoughts or feelings that will move the client forward toward desiring or committing to behavior change.*

Similarly, you wouldn't just throw them in a heap. You would organize the flowers strategically and in a way that emphasizes the beauty of each flower. In the same way, hand pick the client comments that are essential for the client to hear again, and present those "flowers" in an orderly, coordinated manner. However, like flower bouquets, they don't have to be perfect to appear beautiful. Just like when you bring someone flowers, it's the thought that counts.

Points revisited may include specific feelings, ambivalence about change, or even guesses regarding the client's feelings based on verbal and nonverbal communication. Similar to reflections, the practitioner can guess at what the client may be thinking or feeling based on facial expressions or gestures.

While summaries are generally longer than reflections, they are still brief. Refrain from long monologues and pick out only key points that will benefit the client to hear again. In other words, don't allow your bouquet to become overcrowded with weeds.

Summaries don't require an opening line, but at times the following may be used:

> "Let's see if I have it all. . . . "
> "Let's take a step back for a moment and look at all the pieces. . . . "
> "In considering all that you've just told me, it sounds like. . . . "
> "I'm noticing a few themes here. . . . "

It can also help to end a summary with a question such as:

> "How did I do?"
> "Did I get it all?"
> "Did I miss anything? What did I miss?"
> "What else?"

Give the client time to process the summary and respond to the question. Both when reflecting and summarizing, consider the power of silence. Pausing after the client has spoken often prompts the client to talk more, giving important insight into his/her ambivalence. Silences can be uncomfortable and awkward, but necessary, especially for clients who require more time to process. In your responses you naturally set the pace of the discussion. Allow yourself permission to pause, consider, and talk at a speed that is comfortable for both you and the client. It can be easy to get swept away with a stressed-out client who darts here and there, changing topics and going off on tangents. By providing summaries and reflecting your client's body language, you can keep the momentum flowing in the right direction.

SAMPLE SUMMARIES

Here are few examples of summaries provided during a counseling appointment:

> "Let's take a step back for a moment and look at all the pieces. You said you came today because you would like help managing your diabetes and your doctor told you that diet and exercise can help. You

have already made some changes to your eating habits on your own and you're feeling discouraged that while those changes improved your blood sugars, they didn't result in weight loss. I also picked up that losing weight is important to you and I'd like to find out more about that. What is it that you feel losing weight will do for you?"

"It sounds like you have mixed feelings about change. On the one hand, you're excited to start working out more often and have even recently purchased a gym membership. On the other hand, you have voiced a few concerns about working out, mainly a fear of not reaching your goal, your arthritis flaring up, and running out of steam in the evenings, making it hard to get to the gym. We've talked about other times in your life you've been active and you recalled having more energy, sleeping better, and feeling less anxious. What did I miss?"

A more detailed example of piecing together a summary is provided in Figure 9.1.

WHEN TO SUMMARIZE

Really, there's no bad time for a summary. You can offer a bouquet of reflections at any point along the way. Summaries are especially useful during the occasions listed in Figure 9.2.

To Communicate Interest and Understanding

Similar to reflections, summaries demonstrate your interest in understanding what the client is experiencing. And by piecing some key ideas together from the conversation, the client feels as though you are trying to make sense of how the smaller pieces fit together to form a bigger picture. For example:

"When you heard your father tell you to 'go easy on the brownies,' you felt like he was telling you that you needed to lose weight. And it sounds like that made you feel like his love for you was dependent on your appearance or size. You see the connection between those childhood experiences and your current relationship with food and how you see yourself. It's as if your father's voice followed you into adulthood. Did I get it all? How does all that sit with you?"

To Highlight Ambivalence

When you hear the client voice both sustain talk and change talk, it can help to summarize the ambivalence. In doing so, you help the client to

Read the brief excerpt below. As you read, make a mental note of the pieces you hear from the client that you'd like to highlight in the form of a summary.

CLIENT: Since starting the chemotherapy, I have the worst appetite. I try to eat because I know it's important, but the second I smell the food coming from the kitchen, I feel sick.

PRACTITIONER: The smell of food cooking makes it hard and yet you muscle through the nausea because you know it's important to eat.

CLIENT: When I don't eat I get really tired.

PRACTITIONER: You want more energy during the day.

CLIENT: Yeah, I don't want to just sit around and be a chemo zombie.

PRACTITIONER: You want to lead a full life. Finding ways to manage the nausea would help you do that.

CLIENT: I know I can't be at 100% right now and I'm going to have to rest more, but I don't want this cancer to define me.

PRACTITIONER: You're noticing that there might have to be some give and take as you go through chemo. Tell me more about the food piece in this.

CLIENT: I know food gives me energy, I just wish there was some way I could infuse that energy into my body so I didn't have to actually eat it.

PRACTITIONER: Yes, it's hard eating when you just don't feel like it. I bet food has really lost its allure lately.

CLIENT: It has. I used to be a big eater, loved eggs, bacon, cinnamon rolls in the morning. Just ask my wife. She doesn't know what to do with me.

PRACTITIONER: I bet it's been hard for her to see such a drastic change.

CLIENT: Yeah, she's always trying to get me to eat now and before she was always trying to get me to stop eating.

PRACTITIONER: Yes, that's quite a shift. She must really care about you.

CLIENT: Yes, she wants to keep me around.

Key pieces for summary:
- Chemo has resulted in food losing its appeal.
- Kitchen smells trigger nausea.
- Sees food as a way to get energy.
- Doesn't want cancer to take over his life.
- Wants to find ways to manage his nausea.

Practitioner Summary: "Overall, I'm hearing that food has lost its appeal. You're here today because you want to find ways to manage the nausea so that you have more energy. You don't want this cancer diagnosis to define you and if we can figure out the eating piece, it could make all the difference. How does that sound?"

FIGURE 9.1. Piecing together a summary.

become aware of the mixed feelings she has about change. It's best to start with summarizing the sustain talk and end with summarizing the change talk. Leaving the change talk for the end helps move the conversation forward and may evoke additional change talk. For example:

Provide a summary to . . .
- Communicate interest and understanding.
- Transition from one phase of the appointment to another.
- Highlight client ambivalence.
- Reinforce change talk.
- Wrap up a session.

FIGURE 9.2. When to summarize.

"You seem conflicted. You want to avoid the headaches you get when you stop drinking caffeinated beverages, while at the same time you mentioned that you'd like to reduce your reliance on these drinks for energy."

To Reinforce Change Talk

Perhaps the client has recently made several statements indicating an interest in change. You, as the practitioner, would like to summarize the change talk you hear. For example:

"While you still have concerns about the time it takes to buy fresh produce on a regular basis, you have a general interest in trying out the farmers' market. You mentioned that you even looked into the dates, times, and locations of farmers' markets in our area. You've shared that this style of shopping may get you to eat more fruits and vegetables, which you believe might help improve your health in a number of ways. What are some other reasons you can think of to try out the farmer's market?"

To Transition to a New Topic or Phase of the Appointment

You may want to switch gears at several points throughout the appointment. For example, you may be transitioning from the evoking part of the appointment to the planning part of the appointment, or from the engaging process to the focusing process. Perhaps you have a standard list of assessment questions you use at the beginning of each appointment. By summarizing key pieces from the assessment, you can seamlessly transition the client to consider focusing on one behavior change to discuss further. For example:

"Thank you for sharing more details about your current eating patterns. I heard a number of themes we could revisit at some point, if you're interested. First, you shared a general out-of-control feeling around sweet baked goods, especially in the evenings. You also voiced concerns about skipping breakfasts on busy weekdays, and I think I heard an interest in limiting the number of trips you make to the coffee shop for drinks and pastries. It sounds like we could head in a number of directions at this point. What do you already know about diet changes typically made for lowering blood sugars?"

To Wrap Up a Session

Just before the client heads out the door, it may be helpful to revisit some important components of the appointment. These summaries can help remind the client of his or her personal goals and provide an overview of what just happened in the session. For example:

> "As we wrap it up today, let's take a second, if you don't mind, to review the goals you chose. You plan to try out a new physical activity. You are particularly curious about boxing and said that you plan to research some boxing classes in your area and share your findings at our next appointment. Any final thoughts or concerns before you go?"

Once again, there's never really a bad time to provide a summary; just like there's never a bad time to use a full-length mirror instead of a hand-held mirror. In hearing a summary, the client gains perspective and sees the pieces fitting together, ultimately enhancing the counseling experience.

BRINGING THE OARS TOGETHER

Each MI session has a steady rhythm of open-ended questions and reflections. Affirmations and summaries are the unique percussion instruments that are sprinkled throughout the appointment to enhance the overall musical number. Read the following script of a counseling session and notice the gentle rhythm that carries the client along.

> PRACTITIONER: How do you feel about the changes you attempted to make last week? [open-ended question]
>
> CLIENT: You'd be so proud of me! I actually put my fork down in the middle of my meal the other night.
>
> PRACTITIONER: You're excited that you were able to take time to check in with your fullness level during a meal. [reflection]
>
> CLIENT: Yeah, I mean, it was only one time, but I actually decided soon after pausing that I was full for once and didn't clean my plate.
>
> PRACTITIONER: You feel like you were able to break a habit. [reflection]

CLIENT: Yes!

PRACTITIONER: By following through with your goal you've showed yourself that you're committed to making meaningful changes to the way you eat. That is something to feel proud of. [affirmation] What's the next step for you? [open-ended question]

CLIENT: I really need to be more focused during lunch. I eat in front of my computer a lot.

PRACTITIONER: You'd like to try eating mindfully during your lunch hour at work. [reflection]

CLIENT: Yes. At least I would have a cleaner keyboard! You should see the crumbs I shook out of it the other day. That can't be good.

PRACTITIONER: It sounds like you recognize the other potential benefits to eating lunch away from your desk. [reflection]

CLIENT: Yeah—a cleaner computer and desk.

PRACTITIONER: What might make it hard to be more mindful while eating your lunch? [open-ended question]

CLIENT: I don't know, I guess I just feel busy and stressed all the time, like I need to keep working to get it all done in time.

PRACTITIONER: You're more stressed out at work than in other eating environments. [reflection] It sounds like you are quite committed to your work. [affirmation]

CLIENT: Yes, I guess I am, but I'm also just really overworked.

PRACTITIONER: What are other barriers to staying mindful during lunches at work? [open-ended question]

CLIENT: Hmm, I can't think of anything else. I think I'm just in the habit of working while I eat at my desk. If I force myself to just stay in the lunch room when I go pick up my lunch in the office refrigerator, then I wouldn't be as tempted to eat at my desk.

PRACTITIONER: You came up with a solution on your own and that is to eat in the lunchroom. [affirmation] What will your coworkers think? [open-ended question]

CLIENT: Honestly, I don't even think anyone will notice. And if they do, I'll just tell them what we've been working on in these appointments. Maybe it will make them want to try this mindful eating stuff too.

PRACTITIONER: Overall, you're excited about this mindful eating approach and removing distractions while you eat so you can be more aware of your fullness. You were successful at dinner and now you'd like to try eating this way at lunch. You mentioned a concern that you won't have enough time to take a short break to eat your lunch mindfully because you're so busy at work. Not only does taking a lunch break slow down your eating pace so you can tune into how your body feels, but you also mentioned an added bonus of a cleaner workspace and a crumb-free keyboard. You've also figured out a plan, which is to eat your lunch in the break room. [summary]

CLIENT: You know, it's really not that hard to just take a few minutes to eat. I may not be able to do it every day, but I could probably try a few days a week, just to see how I like it.

PRACTITIONER: It sounds like you're interested in setting up another little experiment. [reflection]

CLIENT: Yes. I liked how I didn't feel so stuffed after dinner when I just slowed down the pace and checked my fullness. If I did this at lunch, I wonder if I'd feel less sluggish in the afternoon.

PRACTITIONER: While the cost of 10–15 minutes to take a break and eat your lunch may make you less productive at work, you're wondering if you might have more energy in the afternoon because you won't feel as full or sluggish. [reflection]

CLIENT: Yes, so maybe it will be a wash, in terms of getting work done.

PRACTITIONER: So, let's see—a cleaner workspace, feeling more comfortable, and maybe even more energetic in the afternoon. [summary] Any other benefits of eating a more focused, mindful lunch? [closed-ended question]

CLIENT: Yes. I might actually enjoy the meal!

PRACTITIONER: Good point. [affirmation] It's easy to forget that food is supposed to be fun. Staying mindful might make eating more enjoyable. [reflection] At this point, how motivated are you to eat an undistracted lunch a few days a week on a scale from 0 to 10? Ten means very motivated, and 0 means not at all motivated. [change ruler]

CLIENT: I'd say I'm at a 9.

PRACTITIONER: That's nice and high. Tell me more about why you're a 9. [open-ended question]

CLIENT: Well, I'm realizing there are many benefits to slowing down at lunch and that it may not even cost me any work time in the end, especially if I'm feeling more energetic in the afternoon.

PRACTITIONER: You see the benefits and yet, you aren't quite at a 10. [reflection]

CLIENT: I know there are certain days that it just won't be possible, given my schedule, the stressors at work, or even the social environment.

PRACTITIONER: You're realizing it will be impossible to be perfect with this behavior. [reflection]

CLIENT: Yes, but I can at least improve from what I'm currently doing, which is stuffing my face at my computer.

PRACTITIONER: You're noticing that any movement forward is a step in the right direction. [reflection] I'm wondering if it would be helpful to set a more specific achievable goal for enjoying a more mindful lunch. How many days a week would be reasonable for you? [open-ended question]

CLIENT: I could easily do three weekdays, and at least one weekend day as well.

PRACTITIONER: That seems reasonable. [affirmation] OK, so we have a specific goal to shoot for of three workdays and one weekend day. This would be in addition to the more mindful dinners you've been doing. [summary] At this point, how confident are you that you that you can reach this specific goal on a scale from 0 to 10? [change ruler]

CLIENT: I'm at a 9. I can't say a 10 because I just need to try it first. But, I'm feeling pretty confident now that I've given myself some wiggle room.

PRACTITIONER: You're feeling pretty confident. [reflection] If you take a look at the next few weeks, what barriers, if any, might get in the way? [open-ended question]

CLIENT: Well, I know I have a lunch meeting on Wednesday, so that day is out. On the other days, I guess it's just a matter of remembering.

PRACTITIONER: Can I share with you a technique other clients have tried for remembering a certain behavior? [asking permission question]

CLIENT: Sure.

PRACTITIONER: Some of my clients have found that setting a calendar reminder either on a phone or a computer can help. One idea is that you could set this type of reminder to go off around lunchtime and perhaps write a word that helps you remember the plan such as "mindfulness." [giving information] How does that sound? [open-ended question]

CLIENT: Yes, that will work for me.

PRACTITIONER: Great! Any other barriers that you can think of? [closed-ended question]

CLIENT: Other barriers may come up, but I think I'm at least ready to give it a try.

PRACTITIONER: Changing the way you've done something for so long can be challenging. You've mentioned many reasons you'd like to change the way you eat your meals. We've discussed different strategies that may help you slow down a bit and now you're ready to give them a try. [summary] How would you feel about checking in with one another in 2 weeks? [open-ended question]

CLIENT: That would be great.

PRACTITIONER: Great, we'll see you then.

The script above includes ten open-ended questions, five affirmations, 12 reflections, and four summaries. There were also a few closed-ended questions, and at one point the practitioner provided the client with information. The primary instruments were the reflections and open-ended questions, just like the violins of an orchestra. Like percussion instruments or certain wind instruments, the affirmations and summaries are used less frequently, but bring the music to life. The goal of the orchestra of OARS is to elicit and highlight change talk, thereby moving the client forward in the change process.

PART IV

Beyond the Basics

CHAPTER 10

When Clients Aren't So Sure about Change

> The curious paradox is that when I accept myself just as I am
> then I can change.
>
> —CARL ROGERS

Not every client who walks through your door is going to be ready or willing to change. Appointments are made with nutrition and fitness professionals for a variety of reasons. Sometimes the client initiates the appointment and other times what brings the client in is a physician referral or a nagging spouse. Therefore, it is unrealistic to think everyone who books an appointment with you is ready to start implementing changes right away. However, it doesn't mean that the time you spend with the disinterested client is not valuable.

A skillful practitioner can use certain techniques to guide a client toward change, or at least thinking about change. Just making that initial step, even if only contemplating it, can be a significant accomplishment for someone who was previously not even aware, or who was in denial of the negative consequences of a behavior.

This chapter provides tips and strategies for evoking the internal motivation that is buried even in your least motivated clients.

READING YOUR CLIENT

In the first few seconds of the appointment, you will likely get a good sense of how the client feels about being there. Using both verbal and nonverbal communication, the client sends messages about her interest in change. Crossed arms, furrowed eyebrows and a tilted head would all be strong indicators that a client is angry or disinterested. As she begins to talk, she really starts to express how she feels about the appointment. Much of what the client says about a behavior change can be categorized into three categories: change talk, sustain talk, and discord.

Change talk is anything the client says that favors making a behavior change. Practitioners wish, dream and hope for change talk from their clients, especially the ones that seem disinterested during initial encounters. Change talk sounds like:

> "I really have to figure something out. I can't keep going on and off diets."
> "I hate how much money I spend when I eat out."
> "I'd like to start walking with my friend."
> "I really like yogurt. I didn't think of that. I'd like to try that for breakfast."

Sustain talk is anything the client says that favors not changing. Sustain talk sounds like:

> "I hate sweating."
> "I'm a bit of a picky eater, so this isn't going to be easy."
> "It's so much easier just to eat out for lunch."
> "I'm in too big of a hurry in the morning to eat anything."

Expressing both change talk and sustain talk is a natural part of wading through the waters of ambivalence. Often you'll hear change talk and sustain talk within the same sentence. How you respond to sustain talk and change talk will ultimately determine the client's motivation and interest in making a change. In fact, the way you respond plays a significant role in whether the client remains physically and emotionally present in your office or heads for the door.

The collaborative nature of the counseling relationship is important for creating an environment where the client can focus on motivation and change. A disruption in the relationship between client and practitioner can distract the client from this focus. This disruption is called *discord* between the two parties. Discord sounds like:

> "I already met with a nutritionist and she just told me I had to cut out butter. I don't even eat butter. This is probably going to be a waste of my time just like the last time."
> "What do you eat? You probably eat all perfect, making the rest of us look bad."
> "Send my son to the playground? Are you crazy?! We've got gangs!"
> "You're probably going to tell me I drink too much soda. Everyone's on me about my soda."

Sometimes the client shows up for the appointment angry or resentful and expresses discord before the practitioner has even had a chance to speak. Other times, discord develops as a result of the practitioner moving away from the spirit of MI and is likely to occur if the practitioner starts pressuring the client to change.

> *The collaborative nature of the counseling relationship is important for creating an environment where the client can focus on motivation and change.*

For the most part, discord can be prevented or disarmed through expressing empathy, supporting client autonomy, partnership, and collaboration.

MINIMIZING SUSTAIN TALK AND DISCORD

What's the best way to minimize sustain talk and discord in a session and promote change talk? Communicate in a way that is consistent with the spirit of MI and adjust your counseling style to avoid certain communication snags. When you hear discord, reflective listening works well to defuse hostility. Figure 10.1 includes examples of client discord along with responses that might make matters worse and alternative responses that can turn the conversation in a new direction.

In their first MI book, Miller and Rollnick (1991) named common traps that often increase sustain talk and discord. Those traps, and a few others, are described below along with solutions for steering clear of these pitfalls and staying the course toward client–practitioner harmony.

The Question–Answer Trap

Nutritionist and fitness practitioners have been trained in conducting detailed assessments, complete with a variety of questions about weight and disease history, a dietary or exercise recall, and a slew of other important topics. However, the downside of completing an oral assessment is that the practitioner automatically is placed in the driver's seat, pushing the client into a passive role. The practitioner asks a question, and the client responds to the question. The practitioner asks the next question, and the client responds. This continues on down the line until the assessment is complete. The practitioner is often writing down answers on a clipboard and clients are left wondering what the practitioner is writing and thinking about them.

If peppering clients with questions is not a productive process toward change, then how does the nutritionist or fitness counselor collect this

Client comment	Practitioner response that might *promote* discord	Practitioner response that will likely *reduce* discord
"You're not going to come in here and bug me about not eating enough, are you? The nurses have been nagging me to eat more and I just don't feel like it."	"Actually, I am. Why are you resisting everyone's advice? Don't you know they're just trying to help you get better?"	"Everyone's been pressuring you to eat more and you're really tired of it."
"Don't tell me it's because I drink too much. I've heard that one before and I'm not buying it."	"Yes, alcohol is one thing that raises a person's triglycerides and you did tell me last time that you typically drink four beers a night."	"You think that your triglycerides might be elevated for other reasons. Would it be helpful to talk about those other reasons today?"
"I already paid for this appointment, so you better make it worth my while."	"I'll do my best, but I can't make any promises."	"You are someone who works hard for a living and takes great care to spend your money wisely. You seem worried that I'm not going to be able to help you."
"My last trainer made me work out so hard I threw up and developed shin splints. You're not going to have me pleading for mercy are you?"	"You never know!"	"You're hoping to feel more supported in finding a level of fitness that doesn't result in injury or discomfort. We can definitely work together on that and I hope you'll tell me if you're feeling like I'm pushing too hard."
"I don't know why I have to sit through your lecture every month just to get my food vouchers. You're wasting your time."	"Sorry, that's our policy."	"It sounds like you haven't found our sessions very useful. What could we talk about today that would be more worthwhile?"

FIGURE 10.1. Responding to discord.

important information without putting on the expert hat? Nutrition and fitness practitioners attempting to adopt more MI skills have tried a number of techniques. One strategy is to have the client complete a preappointment questionnaire. The client answers a series of questions in writing before the first appointment. Others have revamped their oral assessments to include more open-ended questions and provide reflective listening statements following each question, to make the assessment more conversational. This technique might keep the client from feeling like he is in the hot seat.

The ultimate goal is to avoid drilling the client with a long list of questions that can make the client feel judged, anxious, and uncomfortable, ultimately decreasing rapport and stifling the counseling relationship.

An Example of the Question–Answer Trap: Practitioner A

PRACTITIONER A: Hello, Janice. My name is Stephanie. Please have a seat. Your doctor has referred you to me because he is concerned about your cholesterol. Let's take a moment and discuss your eating habits. I'd like to look at what you ate yesterday. What did you eat for breakfast?

CLIENT: Yesterday I had a cup of coffee and some cinnamon and brown sugar instant oatmeal around 7.

PRACTITIONER A: The single-serving packages?

CLIENT: Yes, I get the low-sugar ones and just add water.

PRACTITIONER A: OK, how about lunch?

CLIENT: Yesterday we all went out to Mexican food for lunch. I had a chimichanga, rice, and beans.

PRACTITIONER A: Anything to drink with that?

CLIENT: Yes, a Coke.

PRACTITIONER A: OK, how about in between lunch and dinner?

CLIENT: I had a granola bar around 4.

PRACTITIONER A: OK, anything else?

CLIENT: No, just dinner. I had spaghetti with meat sauce and a salad.

PRACTITIONER A: How much pasta did you have?

CLIENT: Maybe a cup of noodles and then ¾ cup of meat sauce.

PRACTITIONER A: And what was in your salad?

CLIENT: I used romaine lettuce; sometimes I use spinach, but I was all out. Then I put cucumber, tomato, some carrots, and Italian dressing.

PRACTITIONER A: OK, would you say yesterday was a typical day for you?

CLIENT: Yes, except we don't always go get Mexican food, but I do usually go out for lunch when I'm at work. You see that's the problem. I eat out a lot I guess. It's just too much in the morning to get lunch together. I've tried it in the past, and I do it for a while, but then I start bringing my lunch and leaving it in the fridge at work. If everyone's going out, then I'm going to go too.

In this dialogue, the client is defending herself and her eating habits. Practitioner A has simply asked what the client ate yesterday, and the client has shifted into a defensive stance. It is possible to shift back to a more MI-style appointment, but it might be less damaging to the client–practitioner relationship to critically evaluate what information is absolutely necessary to help the client. You may not need as many details as you think in order to provide effective counseling.

In an MI appointment, the client is in the driver's seat; therefore the client is going to decide what change she is interested in making regardless of her current patterns. However, there may be a place for some assessment-like questions at the beginning of the appointment, as they may help the client become more aware of areas he or she would like to change. The key is to keep it conversational by asking open-ended questions and reflecting the client's responses. Doing so will minimize the question–answer trap.

Another alternative to a traditional food recall is to invite the client to share perceived dietary strengths and areas for improvement. For example, assessment questions could be tweaked to an open-ended, free-form style such as:

"Tell me about your eating habits."
"What do you think are the positive aspects of your current eating patterns?"
"What do you think are the negative aspects of your current eating patterns?"

When it is necessary to conduct a more formal diet or exercise review, another option is to ask the client to complete a food and exercise record prior to her visit, thereby eliminating the awkward nature of a detailed food and activity recall.

An Example of a More MI-Oriented Assessment: Practitioner B

PRACTITIONER B: Hello, Janice. My name is Stephanie, I'm a nutritionist here in the clinic. Please have a seat. Tell me about yourself and what brings you in today. [open-ended question]

CLIENT: I've lived in this town all my life. I work full-time as a receptionist and have two kids in college.

PRACTITIONER B: Well, great. I look forward to getting to know you today. We have about 30 minutes to talk about anything related to nutrition. So, what would you like to start with? [open-ended question]

CLIENT: Well, I'm here because Dr. Sawyer told me my cholesterol was high. That was about 2 weeks ago. Since then I've been thinking about what I can do. I read somewhere that oatmeal can lower your cholesterol, so I've started eating oatmeal in the mornings. It's been about 3 days that I've been doing that.

PRACTITIONER B: Your conversation with your doctor was a bit of a wake-up call for you and motivated you to make a change on your own. [reflection of change talk]

CLIENT: Yeah, it wasn't that hard. My mom has high cholesterol, so I know a thing or two already.

PRACTITIONER B: And you've seen her make some changes. [continuing the paragraph reflection]

CLIENT: She and my dad changed their diets a lot. I've seen what they've had to do. I think I eat pretty well at breakfast and dinner. It's the lunches that are a problem. Where I work, a core group of us go out to lunch almost every day. We go to Mexican food most often, maybe two to three times a week. Sometimes we go next door to this Chinese place or Thai food. It's a pretty important part of my day.

PRACTITIONER B: You enjoy more than just the food when you go out with them. [reflection]

CLIENT: I have fun with them. If I didn't go, I'd be missing out. But you know, we don't have to go to Mexican or Chinese all the time. A few of them have been complaining that they're gaining weight. My friend Valerie has been bringing her lunch and staying at the office for the last week. I bet she'd really be happy if we stayed in more often. . . .

Practitioner B used reflections and open-ended questions to engage the client, allowing her to talk about what she cares about most. The conversation between the client and practitioner builds a foundation where the client begins to feel comfortable.

Volleying questions and answers back and forth puts the client in a passive role. Another way practitioners tend to take control is to "pounce" on clients by starting a follow-up appointment with something like, "I have your goals from last week here in front of me. Let's see, you said you would work on drinking eight glasses of water a day. How has that been going?" The practitioner's tendency to drive the appointment, however, can be what causes the client to express more sustain talk dismantling a carefully constructed client–practitioner relationship.

The Expert Trap

It is tempting to offer clients unsolicited advice. We all have the urge to tell others what has worked for us. We say things like, "I've been able to get more vegetables in my diet by making soups for dinner. Does that interest you?" or "I've found that parking a few blocks from my office and walking before and after work is an easy way to get exercise in. Would you like to try that?" The problem with the expert trap is that it gives the impression that you are the expert of your client's problem. In actuality, the client is the expert of the client's problem. If the advice giving involves stories from your own life, then you come across as the perfect eater or exerciser. Clients may feel that they cannot disclose certain pieces of information when talking to someone who might not be able to relate to their problems.

An Example of the Expert Trap: Practitioner A

PRACTITIONER A: You know, I've struggled with the same problem you're having now. I just started packing my lunches the night before and bringing them to work with me. I bet that would work well for you since you're so busy in the morning.

CLIENT: I guess so, but I don't know what to pack. I just don't like sandwiches that much.

PRACTITIONER A: Then you should do leftovers or something. It would really help you eat better.

CLIENT: OK. Maybe I'll try that.

PRACTITIONER A: Great, I'll add that to your goal sheet.

Just like with the question–answer trap, giving advice without asking permission and offering choices pushes clients into a passive role. In MI sessions, clients are the experts and the practitioners are there to encourage them to explore their situations and come up with their own solutions. Practitioners help guide clients toward change by finding, exploring, and supporting change talk as well as affirming the qualities that make them able to change. When the time is right, practitioners can also provide specific and targeted information, but this is always done after asking permission from the client.

When you start trying to problem-solve for the client, the client may bear down with sustain talk or simply agree with you because she doesn't want to let you down, but later fail to make the behavior change. As Miller and Rollnick (2013) put it, "motivation for change is not installed, but is evoked" (p. 23).

An Example of Avoiding the Expert Trap: Practitioner B

PRACTITIONER B: You're saying that mornings are busy for you, so packing your lunch in the morning may not be the best time. [reflection] What might work better for you? [open-ended question]

CLIENT: I could probably pack my lunch the night before. I don't know though, sandwiches might get soggy. I actually don't even really like sandwiches. What else could I pack?

PRACTITIONER B: So you're looking for something that won't go bad or get soggy during the day. [reflection] Some clients find that making a little extra for dinner and then packing the leftovers for lunch works. Others have found it's useful to have this list of easy grab-and-go lunch ideas handy. [giving information] I can give it to you if you think it might be useful. [asking permission] It has foods like yogurt, crackers and cheese, hummus and vegetables, or wraps. What are your thoughts on those options? [open-ended question]

CLIENT: Leftovers could work because there is a microwave in our break room. But I don't always have anything left over to pack the next day because my partner is a big eater. I'll probably want to take a look at that list you have also. I like most of the foods you mentioned.

PRACTITIONER B: It's nice to have a back-up plan for when leftovers aren't an option. I also heard you saying that packing your lunch the night before might work better for you than figuring out what to bring in the morning when you're in a hurry. [summary]

In this example, the practitioner simply reflected what the client was saying and used open-ended questions to invite her to come up with a solution. When the client got stuck, the practitioner was there to provide suggestions of foods to pack, referring to ideas that have worked for other clients.

The Scare Tactics Trap

There is a time and place for letting clients know the negative consequences of certain behaviors. However, harping on the dangers of certain negative health choices tends to backfire when clients have low perceptions of self-efficacy or response efficacy. Response efficacy is the belief that the solution provided is not effective in reducing the risk of harm (Witte & Allen, 2000). Scare tactics may not be the answer and they are not consistent with the spirit of MI. When scare tactics are used in health education, the audience can become overwhelmed and immobilized with fear. They turn their focus to coping with their fears with little energy left to focus on behavior change. Furthermore, scare tactics can come across as shaming and rarely result in lifelong behavior change.

An Example of Using Scare Tactics: Practitioner A

"I know you've had a rough first trimester, and you shared that you've had some morning sickness. After reviewing your dietary recall, I'm concerned that your diet is lacking folate. You know if you don't get enough folate in your diet during pregnancy, your baby could have neural tube defects. You really need to eat better."

An Example of Avoiding Using Scare Tactics: Practitioner B

"You've had a rough first trimester. It sounds like you've really been trying to eat a balanced diet and are having a hard time keeping food down. I reviewed your dietary recall and noticed that your diet may be low in folate. What do you know about folate and pregnancy? . . . Would you like to hear more? . . . Folate is an important vitamin for the baby's developing nervous system. What do you make of this information?"

Practitioner B starts with the client. She finds out what the client knows about folate and what concerns the client has. If the client isn't aware of the connection between folate and the developing nervous system, the practitioner is there to provide this piece of information if the client is interested. What cannot be conveyed through this passage is the practitioner's tone of voice. Practitioner B was able to lay the facts on the table but did it in a way that did not frighten or shame the client. This was accomplished with the use of non-inflammatory language while making every effort to remain objective.

The Cheerleading Trap

You mean well when you cheer on your clients. There's no denying you want to see them succeed and that you are proud of them when they make positive health changes. It's one thing to provide encouragement and affirmations, but it's another thing to pull out your pom-poms. Figure 10.2 includes examples of cheerleading statements versus true affirmations.

While the cheerleading statements may sound motivating and encouraging, they can send the client the wrong message. They imply that the client is only successful if he or she makes the change. Consequently, the client may be less likely to share when he or she is struggling. Another negative side effect of cheerleading is that the client may want to make a change only to please you as the practitioner. If that's the case, the client is unlikely to maintain the behavior change long term. Finally, cheerleading can lead to sustain talk rather than change talk. By reflecting one side of a client's ambivalence, it may lead him or her to argue for the other side, thus arguing against changing. Affirmations, on the other hand, are strategically placed to build self-efficacy and intrinsic motivation.

Cheerleading	Affirming
• "You're doing so well!"	• "You care about your health."
• "I'm so proud of you!"	• "Following through with your experiment is really something to feel proud of."
• "Look at you go! I bet those cholesterol numbers are dropping as we speak!"	• "You noticed that you feel better when you eat more fruits and vegetables and that's making you feel like you can do this."
• "You're one of the best clients I've ever had."	• "You found that adding a vegetable to your dinner wasn't too challenging."
• "Keep up the good work!"	• "You feel good about the changes you've been able to make."
• "You did it! You're awesome!"	• "You were successful at coming up with some ways to make this change easy."

FIGURE 10.2. Cheerleading versus affirming.

The Information Overload Trap

There's just so much that you want to tell your clients. You begin thinking, "I may never see this client again; I have to make sure he has all the information he needs." More is better, right? Not when it comes to MI and behavior change. Changing a behavior is hard work. If the client leaves with a long list of changes, it's unlikely he will succeed. Behavior change is typically a product of motivation, not education. Sometimes education is needed for the behavior change to occur, but more often than not, the client already knows which foods are best but isn't able to make the change for other reasons. Find out what the client already knows, and then find out what the client would like to know. Read the client's verbal and nonverbal cues to determine whether he or she is suffering from information overload. If the client begins to look overwhelmed or develops a glazed stare, then you may have gone too far.

> *Behavior change is typically a product of motivation, not education.*

In the section on information exchange (Chapter 5) elicit–provide–elicit (E-P-E) is recommended to avoid information overload. By checking in with what the client knows and asking permission before you provide any information, you are better able to assess the client's needs and then provide relevant and desired information. By ending the information-giving portion with another elicit, you get a chance to assess the client reaction and then decide whether more information is going to be helpful or hurtful.

An Example of Information Overload: Practitioner A

PRACTITIONER A: You have celiac disease, which means you have difficulty digesting and absorbing gluten. Gluten is found in foods containing wheat, barley, and rye. So you're probably wondering what gluten really is. It's actually a compound that's made from two proteins: glutenin and gliadin. When mixed with water and manipulated, these proteins produce an elastic compound that ultimately helps breads rise. Now, when you eat it, your body sees it as a foreign invader and attacks the villi in your small intestine. They collapse and become far less efficient at absorbing food. All of your symptoms are due to this immune response to gluten.

CLIENT: So what does that mean? I can't eat anything.

PRACTITIONER A: So it's bye-bye to bread, pasta, couscous, orzo, most cereals, and flour tortillas.

CLIENT: Well my family is just not going to go for this.

An Example of Offering Information Using E-P-E: Practitioner B

PRACTITIONER B: Your allergy test came back positive for celiac disease. What have you heard of this diagnosis? [open-ended question]

CLIENT: The doctor said I had to follow a gluten-free diet. I'm not sure about this. You hear so much about gluten-free diets recently. I'm just not sure how to go about it.

PRACTITIONER B: You've been thinking about this since you received your lab results and you're overwhelmed with the idea of switching to a gluten-free diet. [reflection]

CLIENT: Yeah, I don't really know where to start.

PRACTITIONER B: There are a few places we could start. Here's a list of topics for celiac disease including "what is gluten" "where is gluten found in foods" "what happens if I eat gluten." Which one, if any, interests you most? [elicit]

CLIENT: OK. Let's start with where gluten is found in foods.

PRACTITIONER B: All right. Gluten is found in wheat, barley, and rye. It can also be found in many oat products. So unless your oatmeal specifies "gluten free" on it, you can assume it's not. [provide] What are you thinking about this information? [elicit]

CLIENT: I didn't realize it was more than just bread. I'm not quite sure I know where those are all hiding in my foods.

PRACTITIONER B: Some of my clients find it helpful to go through this sample menu together and pick out all the foods that have gluten in them. Then I have an alternative gluten-free menu that shows how you can change a few things in order to make it gluten free. Would you like to try this activity? [asking permission]

CLIENT: Yes, that would really be helpful.

Which conversation would you rather have? Practitioner A talks at the client, getting caught up in the science of the disease. Because Practitioner A was so focused on explaining the pathophysiology of celiac disease he was not able to see that the client was getting overloaded with information. Since the information was given without permission or engagement from the client, she responded with sustain talk. Practitioner B, on the other hand, uses an E-P-E technique to offer information and in doing so is able to pick up on how overwhelmed the client was feeling at the beginning of the appointment. By checking in, expressing empathy, and supporting client autonomy by asking her to choose the topics, the practitioner was able to provide the most helpful information. The time spent enhanced the client's learning and she seemed prepared to start voicing change talk.

The Jump-to-Planning Trap

For many practitioners, talking about the "how to" of change is the most enjoyable part. Nutritionists are ready with their quick and easy meal and snack ideas and are eager to pass them along to their clients. Fitness practitioners are eager to start showing their clients certain exercises and resources for community activities. Before diving into the "how to" it's important to spend time engaging and building rapport, exploring ambivalence, and building motivation. Only when the client has expressed a strong desire to change is it time to discuss how the client will proceed. Also, be aware that some clients may seem ready to receive your tips, tricks and strategies, but then respond with sustain talk. A client might sit down and immediately say, "OK, I know I need to eat better. Tell me what to do. Give me a meal plan." This may sound like a clear indication that you should get out a meal plan and start talking about what this person should and shouldn't eat. However, this is a ruse. Although the client is voicing change talk, he or she also wants to take a passive role. It would be helpful to reflect the meaning of this statement and see what the client really wants.

> Only when the client has expressed a strong desire to change is it time to discuss how the client will proceed.

The Chat Trap

Lastly, spending a good amount of time making "small talk" may be a comfortable way to try to build rapport, but it is rarely helpful. Moreover, the flow of the appointment can feel jerky when you decide it's time to get down to business. Building rapport happens through engaging the client in meaningful discussion about what brought him into the appointment. By spending time reflecting and asking open-ended questions, the client gets to know your style and becomes more comfortable talking about important issues with you. Then, as certain themes become more prevalent, you are able to guide him into focusing on some specific areas where change could occur. "Chatting" seems to distract more than it helps.

MI works by finding, exploring, and supporting change talk. However, there will be many instances when clients are not moving toward change, but instead are cementing their positions and arguing for the status quo. Although the client may seem to be the one with the problem, in reality the practitioner may benefit from taking a closer look at his personal communication style. You can't control what the client will say, but you can certainly control what you say and how you say it.

CHAPTER 11

What to Do When There's Little Time

Don't count every hour in the day, make every hour in the
day count.

—UNKNOWN

At first glance, MI may seem like a technique that requires an abundance
of time—time that nutrition and fitness professionals don't often have.
Consider these professionals who are usually short on time:

- A clinical dietitian has received three consults for brief nutrition
  education in addition to 15 initial assessments on the medical/surgi-
  cal floor.
- A personal trainer wonders how to fit MI into a session that also
  includes teaching the client a series of exercises.
- A public health nutritionist has 15-minute sessions with each client
  before providing food vouchers.
- A physical therapist talks to her client about how his exercises are
  going at home while he warms up for 5 minutes on the stationary
  bike.

This chapter homes in on the key essentials of MI and describes how
to maintain the spirit of MI even when interactions with clients are short.
While MI may take a little longer than lecturing a client, consider the cost
of *not* using it. Without engaging the client and evoking change talk, the
odds that the client will attempt a change are slim. Failure to assess readiness to change and ask permission before giving information may result in
defensiveness and might reduce motivation. The cost of not spending those
few extra seconds to maintain the spirit of MI results in a client tuning you
out and putting you on the list of "I tried that once and it didn't work."

Consider the following example of a nutrition practitioner who is in a hurry and decides she doesn't have time for MI:

PRACTITIONER: Hi, Mrs. Wilson, I'm Natalie. I'm a dietitian. Your doctor asked that I stop by to tell you about the right diet for chronic kidney disease.

CLIENT: You mean I actually have a disease? The doctor told me my kidneys weren't looking too healthy, but he didn't say anything about a disease. Gosh. How long do I have to live?

PRACTITIONER: Yes, technically your condition is called chronic kidney disease, but don't worry, some people have this condition for years. I have a handout here with a few basic dos and don'ts for patients with kidney disease. Why don't you take a look? (*Gives the patient the handout.*) As you can see, the most important thing you can do is control your blood sugars and blood pressure so that your kidneys don't get worse. I saw on your chart that your issue is blood pressure. So be sure to follow the diet for blood pressure—you know, reduce salt, eat more fruits and vegetables, that kind of thing. It's important to increase your activity too. Do you have any questions?

CLIENT: I don't know. I've been keeping the salt shaker off the table, so that's at least one thing.

PRACTITIONER: Yes, that's a good start, but there's also a lot of sodium in food, so be sure to read your food labels too.

CLIENT: Right, I remember being taught that by my nutritionist. I remember to do that sometimes in the grocery store. I couldn't believe how much sodium was in the frozen chicken nuggets I usually get for my grandkids to eat after school.

PRACTITIONER: It adds up quickly. It's important to always check.

CLIENT: I know, I know. I'll try to be better about that.

PRACTITIONER: Good. You can also control your blood pressure by eating more fruits and vegetables and being more physically active.

CLIENT: Yes, I eat pretty well. I always have a banana in the morning and some sort of salad at dinner.

PRACTITIONER: Good, that's a start. And are you exercising regularly?

CLIENT: Well, not really that often. I may get out and go shopping once in a while, but that's about it.

PRACTITIONER: Consider getting something more regular started, like taking a short walk in the morning while it's cooler.

CLIENT: I know I need to. I don't like walking by myself. It's boring and I'm always worried something bad is going to happen. Have you watched the news lately? Just awful!

PRACTITIONER: Yes, you're right, safety is important. Well, maybe you can find a friend to go with you. I have to go now, but I'd like to schedule you an appointment to see a dietitian next time you see your regular doctor. I'll just leave this handout for you to look at when you get home. Take care, Mrs. Wilson!

Now consider the dietitian who is short on time but chooses to use MI anyway:

PRACTITIONER: Hi, Mrs. Wilson, I'm Natalie. I'm a dietitian. Your doctor asked that I come in to talk to you about your kidneys. Would that be OK with you if we chatted for a few minutes? [asking permission]

CLIENT: Sure, that's fine. I've met with a nutritionist before and I know what I've got to do.

PRACTITIONER: What do you already know about good nutrition for healthy kidneys? [eliciting what the client knows before providing information]

CLIENT: Well, I don't know about kidneys, I just remember being told I couldn't eat so much salt.

PRACTITIONER: You're right; limiting salt can help you control your blood pressure, and controlling your blood pressure is a great way to keep your kidneys healthy. Would you be interested in taking a look at this handout I have on other strategies for keeping kidneys healthy? [asking permission]

CLIENT: Yes, go ahead and put that on my chair with those other discharge papers.

PRACTITIONER: Sure, I can do that. Hearing about your kidneys yesterday must have felt a bit worrisome. [expressing empathy] It may make you feel better to hear that by eating well and being active, you can slow down how fast your kidneys lose their function. [giving information]

CLIENT: Yes, that is good news, I guess. It's nice to feel like there's something you can do about it. [change talk—ability to change] But at the same time, I've never done all that great on the diets I've tried. [voicing ambivalence]

PRACTITIONER: On the one hand you're apprehensive about making changes to your diet and on the other hand you're interested in maintaining your kidney function for as long as possible. [double-sided reflection of the ambivalence]

CLIENT: That's right! I'd like to at least try.

PRACTITIONER: I'm wondering today with this news regarding your kidneys from your doctor, how interested are you in trying to make a change in your eating habits or physical activity on a scale from 0 to 10, where 10 is very interested and 0 is not at all interested? [assessing readiness to change]

CLIENT: OK. Oh, I guess at about a 6.

PRACTITIONER: You're on the fence about it right now, and yet you didn't choose a 4 or a 5. What made you pick a number just on the other side of the fence? [open-ended question to evoke change talk]

CLIENT: Well, I guess I'm just a little worried about my kidneys. I'd really like to keep them healthy, so I'd like to think that this time will be different. [change talk—reason to change]

PRACTITIONER: This new diagnosis has you motivated to do things to take care of your health. [reflecting change talk] If you'd like, I can schedule you to see our outpatient dietitian in a month when you return to see your doctor. How would you feel about that? [asking permission]

CLIENT: Yes, that's a good idea.

PRACTITIONER: Before I leave, I'm wondering if you can think of a time you were successful in making a change that you were able to sustain. [open-ended strengths-based question]

CLIENT: I did end up taking the salt shaker off the table after the last time I met with the nutritionist and it's still off. I do salt my food a little when I'm cooking it, but before I was salting it in the kitchen and at the table.

PRACTITIONER: You were able to make a change you felt good about and you've stuck with it. [affirmation] Making small gradual changes over time can really make a difference. If you were to make another small change to support your kidney health, what would it be? [focusing question that emphasizes autonomy]

CLIENT: I'm thinking I can just throw the salt shaker out altogether at some point. I got used to the food with less salt last time and I can get used to it again. [change talk—ability to change]

PRACTITIONER: You noticed that while your food tasted different at first, you adapted after you gave it some time. [reflecting change talk]

CLIENT: Yes, it's just a matter of throwing it in the garbage, so I won't be tempted.

PRACTITIONER: It sounds like getting the salt out of the kitchen will make it easier for you to make the change you intend to make. Well, I have to go now, but it was nice meeting you, Mrs. Wilson.

While incorporating MI took a little more time, the client in the second interaction has a much higher chance of making a change. The extra minutes spent are sure to pay off. There were a few key MI techniques the practitioner used during that brief interaction.

The dietitian:

- Expressed interest in what the client had already learned previously.
- Used consistent reflections that highlighted change talk.
- Assessed readiness to change using a change ruler.
- Asked about previous successes and affirmed the client's efforts.
- Asked permission before providing information.
- Demonstrated autonomy by inviting the client to consider one small change to focus on at home.
- Expressed confidence that the client would be successful at making a change when she was ready.

SHORTENING THE MI PROCESS

The four processes of MI—engage, focus, evoke, and plan—provide structure to an MI session. (These four processes are covered in depth in Chapters 3–5.) It may take an MI practitioner several sessions before all four processes are covered, or only a few minutes. Timing depends on the client's readiness to change and the practitioner's availability.

If the client is expressing sustain talk or a general lack of interest in making a behavior change, then it may be several sessions before he or she is ready to discuss tips and strategies for change. In that case, a practitioner who is short on time could offer brief interactions that revolve around exploring ambivalence and evoking change talk. Alternatively, if a client is expressing significant change talk and seems ready to discuss change strategies, then shorter sessions that emphasize the planning process may be sufficient.

If client interactions at your workplace must be brief, you may be looking for the bare essentials of the four processes. Below are strategies for shortening each process, if time is limited.

While you may be pressed for time, it's still important to display the same warmth, compassion, and attentive listening.

Engage

It's tempting to jump into planning when time is limited. While you may not have time to explore the client's back story with the leisurely pace of an hour's visit, it's still important to display the same warmth, compassion, and attentive listening. Some busy practitioners find that it's best to avoid questions like, "How are you feeling?" or "How are you?" because they tend to result in answers that fail to assist much in building rapport and take the client in an unproductive direction. Instead use the time you do have to practice thoughtful, complex reflections that represent the true and intended meaning within your client's statements. Engaging is not a process that begins and ends, but is clearly felt throughout your client interactions as you build a working relationship together.

Focus

When you have little time, the focusing process becomes essential. Invite your client to select just one behavior change area he'd like to explore further. Here is a short script from a physician who would like to address health behaviors but has little time to do so.

> PRACTITIONER: Unfortunately, we only have about 5 minutes today. Which, if any, of these topics interest you as an area you may want to work on? *(Gives the client a handout with topics including nutrition, fitness, smoking cessation, stress management, and sleep.)*
>
> CLIENT: I know I need to work on my diet and get more exercise.
>
> PRACTITIONER: You'd like to make changes in your eating and activity levels. [reflection] Which would be more realistic for you to address right now? [focusing]
>
> CLIENT: Probably fitness. I probably need more help with that than you can give me in 5 minutes.
>
> PRACTITIONER: Making a change in your activity level seems simpler. [reflection]
>
> CLIENT: Not easy, but at least easier than changing my food habits.

Clients like to have choices. However, if there is one particular behavior you're required to inform the client about, give the client autonomy in deciding how he might go about making that change. For example, perhaps you are required by your supervisor to talk to your client about reducing the amount of soda he

When you have little time, the focusing process becomes essential.

drinks. You can still give him several different strategies for cutting back on soda and invite him to select a strategy that might work for him. Of course, in the spirit of autonomy, make it clear to the client that not reducing his soda intake at all is always an option.

Evoke

If time is limited, and you only have time for a few open-ended questions that evoke change talk, consider using a change ruler. By asking the client his readiness to change on a scale from 0 to 10, you'll receive a concise response that gives you a good indication of his level of ambivalence. Follow up change ruler questions with probing questions that elicit change talk such as, "You're at a 7, which tells me you have some hesitations, but you're not at a 5 or 6, so what led you to choose a higher number?" Another essential question for evoking change talk is, "In what ways will making this change make your life better?" By encouraging the client to talk about what matters most in making this change, she will come to realize her internal motivators.

When time is limited, it may be tempting to ignore extensive sustain talk from a client and move into the planning process before she is ready. You may find that when you begin discussing possible strategies for change with the client, she is unable to come up with viable solutions and expresses disinterest in every option you provide. This is one sign that the client is not ready for change and it may be worthwhile to return to the evoking process and invite her to convey possible negative consequences of not making a change. In future sessions you could include topics such as her meaning of health and wellness, life goals and values, and social support.

Regardless of your client's readiness to change, summarizing change talk after asking some key evoking questions can help the client move forward. In addition, summaries provide a seamless transition if the client is ready to move into discussing how he might go about making a change. A brief summary sounds like this:

> "You've been living with HIV for a long time and recently started the anti-retroviral therapy. You're finding it challenging to keep up with all the pills and suggested meal timing for the different medications. You understand the importance of being consistent with your medications for keeping your immune system healthy and would like to make a change in this area as long as you can stay within your food budget."

Plan

A simple acronym developed by David B. Rosengren (2009) can help you remember how to assist the client in the planning process when there is little time: FOCUS.

- First ask permission. Asking permission only takes a second and is essential in creating a partnership between the practitioner and client where the client feels in charge and respected.
- Offer ideas. Within a brief MI session, ideas are offered with permission and ideally after eliciting ideas from the client.
- Concise. When offering ideas, keep explanations brief. Also refrain from offering too many ideas at once.
- Use a menu. If you only offer one or two ideas, you limit the chance that the client will find the idea acceptable. By offering a menu of options for how to make a change, the client is more likely to find a solution that works for him.
- Solicit what the client thinks. After providing information or a list of options for making the change, use an open-ended question to gauge the client's interest.

The four processes of MI do not have to be lengthy to serve their purpose. In fact, if the client is expressing readiness to change, then these four processes may be covered in less than 10 minutes. An outline of a brief session that covers the four processes of MI is provided in Figure 11.1.

SIX STRATEGIES TO MI-INSPIRED SESSIONS

MI concepts can be incorporated into a client interaction with minimal effort and significant pay off. If you don't have time for a full session, here are six strategies for making your current interactions more consistent with MI.

1. Narrow the Focus

There are many changes that *could* be made, but likely only one or two changes that the client *would like* to make. Determine the focus from the beginning of the session by agenda mapping to help the client choose. For example:

> "There are many changes we could talk about today that could help your daughter eat a wider variety of foods. Can I share a few directions we could take? [Wait for client response.] We could discuss fun ways to cut and serve fruits and vegetables, strategies for sneaking them into meals or snacks, or what to say at mealtimes that can eliminate the power struggle. Which of these ideas, if any, would be useful?"

2. Take Every Opportunity to Affirm

It's amazing what a little affirmation can do to increase the client's self-efficacy, boost self-confidence, or defuse discord. For example:

Engage
- Introduce self and role.
- "What brings you in today?"
- "What were you hoping to get out of this appointment?"
- Summarize and let the client know the allotted time for the appointment.

Focus
- "If it's all right with you, I have a sheet of paper with different changes that clients often make. What jumps out at you, if anything, as a change you might be interested in making?"

Evoke
- "Why did you select that particular change?"
- "How would that change make your life better?"
- "How interested are you in making that change on a scale from 0 to 10, with 0 being not at all interested and 10 being very interested? Why did you select that number?"
- Reflect and summarize change talk.

Plan
- "How might you go about making that change?"
- "Would you be interested in hearing other strategies that have worked for clients attempting to make that same change?"
- Offer ideas.
- "Which of these strategies, if any, interest you?"
- "How do you see that fitting into your life?"
- "How confident are you that you can make that change on a scale from 0 to 10, with 0 being not at all confident and 10 being very confident? Why did you select that number?"
- "What might keep you from following through with your plan? What ideas do you have for overcoming those barriers?"
- Summarize change talk, highlighting the client-selected behavior change.

FIGURE 11.1. The four processes of MI when there is limited time.

"It's really amazing how you've been able to care for your daughter even with the postpartum depression and limited sleep you've been able to get because of the new baby."

3. Ask Permission before Providing Information

By asking permission before providing information, you express autonomy and partnership, key components of the MI spirit. For example:

"Would it be OK if I gave you some different recipes that were big hits with other children?"

4. Check In

It's important to check in with the client frequently throughout a session to maintain engagement and demonstrate partnership. To avoid lecturing your client or long monologues filled with excessive information, break it up into shorter segments by sandwiching important information between two open-ended questions. (See elicit–provide–elicit in Chapter 5.)

"What strategies have you already tried to encourage your daughter to eat a variety? [elicit] Would you be interested in hearing other ideas? [asking permission] Researchers have found that pressuring children to eat certain foods is rarely effective; what seems to be more helpful is serving the disliked foods repeatedly using different cooking techniques, sauces, and toppings. It's also useful to make sure the child is hungry before the mealtime. Children are much more likely to try new foods when they are hungry, so spacing out meals and snacks is important. [provide] What do you think about all of that? [elicit]

5. Encourage Client-Centered Goal Setting

The client is going to feel more empowered to change if she selects her own goals. By inviting her to set her own goals, you put the client in charge. She knows what works for her life. For example:

"With all that we've talked about today, is there a specific tip or strategy you'd like to try when feeding your daughter? When would you like to try that? How often?"

6. Address Possible Barriers

Before your client leaves the office, offer the opportunity to troubleshoot. For example:

"How confident are you on a scale from 0 to 10 that you can be successful at making the change you've decided on? What might get in your way?"

These six strategies are demonstrated in the script below of a brief interaction between a personal trainer and his client at the YMCA.

PRACTITIONER: I know of a few exercises that you can do that won't bother your knees. Would you be interested in hearing those? [strategy 3, ask permission]

CLIENT: Sure. I know running is bad on your knees.

PRACTITIONER: Yes, running can be hard on your knees. Exercises that are easier on your joints include swimming, aqua jogging, water aerobics, and walking. Using the elliptical machine might also work, but you'd have to test it out. Which, if any, of these activities appeal to you? [strategy 1, narrow the focus]

CLIENT: I'm not much of a swimmer, and I can't really see myself joining my wife's water aerobics class, but I could try aqua jogging while she's in her class. How does that work, exactly? I mean, I could do that in the shallow end, but that might get boring after a while.

PRACTITIONER: That's true. They make these floating devices that you wear like a belt and they keep you buoyant in the water so that you can continue the running motion in the deep end while staying afloat. I'd be happy to show you at your next session. If you're interested, you could bring your swimsuit and you can try out my aqua jogging belt to see if you like it. What do you think about that idea? [strategy 4, check in]

CLIENT: Yes, I'd like to do that. [change talk—activation]

PRACTITIONER: Aqua jogging sounds like something you'd like to try. [reflecting change talk] If you do find that you enjoy aqua jogging, how many days a week do you think you'd be interested in fitting that into your schedule? [strategy 5, encourage client-centered goal setting]

CLIENT: Well, I can definitely do it the two days a week my wife is doing her water aerobics class. [change talk—activation]

PRACTITIONER: You're thinking that at the very least you'll be able to do it 2 days a week since she'll be doing her class at the same time. [reflecting change talk] What, if anything, might get in the way of you following through with your plan? [strategy 6, address possible barriers]

CLIENT: The weather. Since it's an outdoor pool, I'm sure I won't feel like going in the winter. I've always admired my wife for sticking with her water aerobics class in the winter, but I'm not nearly as disciplined as she is.

PRACTITIONER: While you're committed to staying active in the winter, [strategy 2, affirm] you'd like to find something that's a little warmer on those cold, rainy days.

CLIENT: Yeah, while my wife is out in the cold, I'll be in here walking on the treadmill.

PRACTITIONER: You thought of your own alternative that easily aligns with your wife's schedule and seems more enjoyable in the winter months. [strategy 2, affirm]

While this brief interaction between a personal trainer and client may not have all the pieces of a complete MI session, certain strategies were implemented to support client autonomy while still providing some guidance and direction. As a result, the client felt supported and empowered to attempt a new activity.

COMMUNICATING WITH A TALKATIVE CLIENT

While encouraging clients to talk about a behavior change is an essential component of MI, an overly talkative client can make it challenging to promote change talk and set goals while still staying on schedule. Here are a few strategies that allow you to remain an active, caring, and compassionate listener while supporting behavior change.

Reflective Listening and Summaries

By providing concise reflections and summaries, you demonstrate that you care about your client and wish to understand her motivators and barriers surrounding making a change. In addition, you can pull different pieces of what the client says together to help keep the conversation on topic and moving forward. In this example, the client is off in many directions and the practitioner reflects the change talk instead of the tangent.

> PRACTITIONER: Describe a time when you've been successful in the past with making a change.
>
> CLIENT: I started training for a half marathon one time. I did the whole thing—joined a running group, started out slowly, bought new shoes; I really went for it. But then I got shin splints after about 10 weeks of training and had to stop. I felt like such a failure. My brother was doing it with me and he was able to do the whole thing. I was totally jealous. But that pretty much sums up our relationship. He's been beating me out my whole life—he got better grades, did better in sports, dated cute girls, and the list goes on. For once, it felt like we weren't competing, but doing something together and cheering one another on. And my body just couldn't handle it. I had to sit on the sidelines and cheer him on, which was fun, but I really wanted to be out there with him.
>
> PRACTITIONER: If it weren't for the injury, you would have been right there with him. You were committed and excited about the change you were trying to make.

By picking out the intention to change and presenting it, you encourage the client to speak more about it. If the practitioner had instead reflected the feelings of failure or inadequacy, the conversation would have taken a different direction.

Refocusing

It's easy for clients to start talking, and before you know it, you're off in a new direction. A refocusing statement can help guide the client back on track or navigate in a new direction, depending on the client's preference. In this example, the practitioner assists a client struggling with unintentional weight loss.

> PRACTITIONER: From the handout we went over with tips for boosting calories, you chose adding supplemental nutrition shakes between meals as the change you'd like to make. How would your life be better if you made the commitment to drinking those on a regular basis?
>
> CLIENT: I'm sure I'd have more energy. And my son would stop telling me that I look sick. He's been trying to make me different foods that are loaded with butter and sour cream. He's a good cook. I appreciate his help. I try to think of ways I can do that, but I'm not as creative in the kitchen. I tried adding fats to the foods I cooked and it just turned out greasy and unappealing. The other day I drowned my salad in dressing because I knew I needed the extra calories, and it ruined my salad—made it wilted and soggy.
>
> PRACTITIONER: Yes, we could talk about cooking ideas for boosting calories. Which topic would you prefer to talk about first—supplemental drinks or ways to boost calories in your favorite recipes?
>
> CLIENT: We can stick with the drinks for now. That change seems easier to make.
>
> PRACTITIONER: OK, you mentioned that adding supplemental drinks between your meals would give you more energy and get your son off your back.

In this example, the client first voiced interest in adding between-meal nutrition shakes to boost calories and then expressed interest in a different change of adding more dietary fat to meals. While both changes are possible, it's best to assist the client with one change at a time. The practitioner noticed the topic shifting and provided a refocusing response to invite the client to determine the best direction for the session.

Breaking in with Kindness and Compassion

When doing MI, it's best to refrain from interrupting clients and fight the temptation to finish their sentences. However, when working with extremely talkative clients, it may be necessary to break in now and then. A polite way to intercede is to ask permission and voice your timeline.

> CLIENT: . . . and then I told him that he has to go bowling with me because he has to get out of the house. The man never leaves the house except to get the mail. He sits around all day and watches TV and . . .

> PRACTITIONER: If I may jump in for just a moment, I'm concerned we're not going to be able to discuss the reason your doctor asked me to see you. Unfortunately, we only have about 10 minutes today and I want to make sure I have time to answer any questions you have about controlling your blood sugars. If it's OK with you, I'd like to show you a list of changes clients often make to improve blood sugar control. Then perhaps you could select an area you'd like to talk more about. How does that sound?

Giving the client an indication of the amount of time available may leave the client more mindful of the length of his or her responses. In the example, the practitioner makes it clear that he cares about his client and that it's in the client's best interest to keep the conversation on topic. This subtlety may not work with everyone, and for those extra-talkative clients, break in with what you see happening: "Janice, I'm having a hard time following you. If you wouldn't mind, maybe we could slow down for a minute. You have a lot on your mind. What do you feel is the greatest challenge to controlling your blood sugars?" A statement like this one still allows the client to drive, just not in circles.

Clients are going to do more talking as a result of MI, especially with strategically placed open-ended questions and reflections. However, both are essential in evoking change talk and ultimately awakening the client's motivation. The key to short sessions is providing concise, mobilizing reflections and summaries that keep the conversations moving forward.

Even in the shortest interactions, the practitioner can maintain the spirit of MI by implementing a few key skills such as guiding the client to come up with his own goals, asking permission before providing information, and affirming him when opportunities arise. While these strategies may take a few extra minutes, they are worth every second when the result is a more motivated client.

The key to short sessions is providing concise, mobilizing reflections and summaries that keep the conversations moving forward.

CHAPTER 12

Clarifying Health Misinformation and Exploring Unhealthy Beliefs

The most confused we ever get is when we try to convince
our heads of something our hearts know is a lie.
—KAREN MONING

Health information is everywhere. Health is interesting not only to each of us, but also to the advertisers and marketing experts who want to capitalize on any perceived health problems. Prescription and over-the-counter drug companies benefit by making people think there is something wrong with them that they can cure, alleviate, or treat. Commercial weight-loss programs want people to think they are overweight and out of shape, so the purveyors of those programs can serve up a unique solution . . . for a fee, that is.

There is no shortage of health information, both credible and ridiculous, available to consumers. This chapter discusses MI techniques to use when guiding clients who know just enough health-related information to get themselves into trouble. In addition, this chapter focuses on unhealthy beliefs about food, exercise, and body image that emerge from incorrect or outdated information, and how common MI techniques can be used to help clients move toward making sustainable changes that enhance health.

Standing in the checkout line in the grocery store provides a telling example of the onslaught of health information one receives each day. Celebrity weight-loss secrets glare up at us, cooking magazines display delightful pictures of healthy meals on the cover, and TV doctors seemingly stare straight at us, beside the comment "IS YOUR CHOLESTEROL TOO HIGH?" The truth is, we have access to a large amount of good and bad information when trying to manage our own health. It's difficult, even as health professionals, to be completely immune to the subtle influences of this mix of credible and completely inaccurate information. Therefore, the

175

question is how do you help clients weed through the mess of misinformation without making them feel judged or belittled?

Some health professionals take it personally when clients ask questions about fad diets or show attachment to certain diet rules not based on sound science. In these situations, it's tempting for the health professional to scoff at the behavior. He or she may say something like, "That doesn't make any sense" and expect the client to dismiss the diet or product and move on to something more productive. Although the client may say nothing, he ends up feeling embarrassed and judged, and just when he was really beginning to like and trust his nutrition counselor.

There are so many possible topics to discuss in nutrition and fitness counseling. From the very beginning, clients are sometimes apprehensive about what they will be asked to change. An MI practitioner isn't going to prescribe certain lifestyle changes because it forces the client into a passive role in the behavior change process, but the client may not be aware of that in the beginning. Instead, the practitioner is going to elicit what the client is interested in exploring, what information gaps may be present, or what specific problems the client is struggling with. Therefore, the practitioner walks alongside the client and gently guides him or her through ambivalence and toward change.

It's important to be mindful of your own agenda when first entering an appointment. Letting go of your own agenda isn't the same as having no focus or direction within the process of change; quite the contrary. However, with every client, you enter into a partnership where your role is to see the problem through the eyes of the client, rather than through your own.

A guiding style allows both the practitioner and the client to negotiate the agenda. If the client is misinformed about a topic, she likely is unaware that her facts are incorrect. Clarifying the misinformation will understandably not be one of her goals for the appointment. When using a guiding style, the practitioner prioritizes what the client wants to talk about and may offer clarification for the misinformation voiced by the client.

You may detect beliefs based on misinformation within the first few minutes of a session. If you respond by immediately correcting the client you may set the stage for increased sustain talk and discord. While he or she may be impressed with your knowledge of the scientific literature, you also risk coming across as arrogant and unapproachable. Here are some strategies for correcting misinformation while at the same time emphasizing client autonomy.

You may detect beliefs based on misinformation within the first few minutes of a session. If you respond by immediately correcting the client you may set the stage for increased sustain talk and discord.

RESISTING THE RIGHTING REFLEX

The righting reflex is the temptation to provide unsolicited advice or information that corrects something perceived as wrong in the client's statement. It's important to tame the righting reflex when you hear misinformation and instead respond with compassion, respect, and an overall sense of curiosity. Consider the following interactions. The first dialogue showcases Practitioner A, a diabetes educator. He starts off on the right track but is thrown off course when he hears the client voice incorrect nutrition information.

> PRACTITIONER A: What do you typically drink? How do you stay hydrated?
>
> CLIENT: I usually drink juice. Juice doesn't have sugar in it. It's natural.
>
> PRACTITIONER A: Oh no. Where did you hear that? Juice may have natural sugar, but it's still sugar. The first thing I want you to do when you get home is to throw out the juice. Do you think you can do that?
>
> CLIENT: I don't know.

The urge to quickly and concisely correct clients may surface when you hear them repeat incorrect information. You may believe it is your duty to correct misinformation and provide advice. With MI, however, the purpose is not to give advice. The purpose is to cultivate change. Practitioner A may have fulfilled *his need* to provide information but he will be woefully ineffective at meeting the needs of the client.

Alternatively, Practitioner B is not caught off guard when hearing misinformation. He remembers to reflect and ask permission before providing a small amount of information, and then checks in with the client.

> PRACTITIONER B: What do you typically drink? How do you stay hydrated? [open-ended question]
>
> CLIENT: I usually drink juice. Juice doesn't have sugar in it. It's natural.
>
> PRACTITIONER: It's important to you to make food choices that improve your health and well-being. [affirmation] I wonder if it'd be helpful if we talked a little about sugar and where it's found in foods. [asking permission]
>
> CLIENT: OK.
>
> PRACTITIONER B: Sugar comes in many forms. It can be in the form of table sugar or corn syrup, and it can also be less visible. Fruit contains a natural form of sugar that is also found in juice. In 100% fruit juice the sugar is not processed or added, but it still

greatly affects one's blood sugar. [provide] What do you make of this information? [elicit]

CLIENT: I didn't realize that.

PRACTITIONER B: Considering this information, I wonder if the juice you're drinking is driving your blood sugars up. What do you think? *[Elicit]*

Practitioner B has a much better chance of influencing the client because of the respectful manner in which she communicates. By asking permission and eliciting how the client responds to the information, the practitioner supports client autonomy. The practitioner prioritizes the client's needs over her own.

PROVIDING INFORMATION USING ELICIT–PROVIDE–ELICIT

People have all sorts of beliefs about food, how to eat, when to eat, and what to eat. These types of food-related beliefs have been passed down from one generation to another since the beginning of humanity and change as life's circumstances change. Many beliefs about food and eating come from the caregivers in a family. Mothers and grandmothers have a particular impact on one's eating habits. "Always eat your vegetables" or "Clean your plate" are common phrases at the dinner table. Some of this advice is helpful; some is not.

In addition to caregivers, food and eating advice comes from people of perceived authority in health and wellness. Doctors, health coaches, and anyone who publishes a book on the subject have an impact on what people believe about food. Nutritionists are constantly asked which diet rules are fact and which are fiction. Entire TV shows are dedicated to issuing food rules to help people lose weight or cure ailments. The principles of information exchange from Chapter 5 apply when correcting false information. Elicit–provide–elicit (E-P-E) is a useful tool for gently pointing clients in the right direction.

Elicit

Elicit before providing information contrary to what the client thinks. The purpose is to gain permission, assess prior knowledge, or gauge overall concerns or interests in the topic. In the previous scenario about juice, the practitioner first asks permission before talking about where sugar is found:

"It's important to you to make food choices that improve your health and well-being. [affirmation] I wonder if it'd be OK with you if I talk a little about sugar and where it's found in foods. [asking permission]"

In another scenario, the practitioner assesses the client's knowledge about foods high in sodium by asking an open-ended question in a non-judgmental way:

"You have been trying to control your blood pressure by eating less salt. What kinds of foods strike you as being particularly high in salt?"

In the next scenario, the practitioner assesses the client's concerns about diet pills before providing information:

"You're interested in taking the diet pills your mother gave you. What concerns do you have, if any, about taking them?"

This last scenario gauges the client's interest level by using an agenda-mapping exercise to focus the conversation:

"You've mentioned a few things this morning and I wonder which is more important to you to talk about today. Earlier, you said you've been making your son, Sam, whole-grain breakfast pastries in the morning because they're fast, he likes them, and you're thinking the whole grain makes them a good breakfast. I could offer you some healthy, quick breakfast ideas if it would be useful to give you a little variety. You've also said that you're concerned about your son overeating when he is at his dad's house and he seems to be making unbalanced snack choices in the afternoon. Which, if any, of these topics would you like to focus on today?"

Before providing any information to a client, whether it is novel or clarifying, harness the spirit of MI and first ask permission. Remember, it is completely within your client's right to refuse this information. A refusal may not be a straightforward "no" but simply a shift to a different subject, or the client may speak as if you hadn't said anything at all. Take these subtle hints as a polite way of saying, "No thank you, I'd rather keep talking about this now."

Provide

As with usual information exchange, clarifying health misinformation requires the practitioner to lay important groundwork before providing information. Once that's done, though, it's time to share the information you have with your client. Here are four tips to keep in mind when providing information.

Provide Only Relevant Information

The client gave you permission to talk about a specific topic, not to ramble on or shift to another topic entirely. Stay on topic and only provide information that is relevant to the situation. Health practitioners have a tendency to tell their personal experiences as a way of relating to and motivating their clients. Especially in health counseling, it's common to find practitioners who have struggled and succeeded with their own health challenges.

Self-disclosure can be a powerful way to tell clients they are not alone and you truly understand their challenges on a personal level. However, it can easily switch gears into a conversation about the practitioner and not the client. If you decide self-disclosure is appropriate, keep it relevant to the client's issue and make every effort to see the circumstance through the eyes of client and not through your own experience. Just because your experience was similar does not mean it is the same.

Keep It Short

Information overload can happen when a practitioner monopolizes the conversation. Although it may be pertinent, clients become disengaged when the practitioner becomes long winded in her explanation. Focus on clear and concise explanations that engage the client.

Use Understandable Terms

Medical terminology was developed for practitioners to easily communicate with one another. Latin root words are further described with prefixes and suffixes that fully explain the treatment, procedure, disease, or condition. Although useful in the medical field, medical terminology has a way of dismantling the client–counselor relationship by making the counselor assume the expert role. Medical terminology belongs in the client's medical chart, not in the information exchange between client and practitioner. Support the client's role as the expert by using commonly understood words, such as those listed in Figure 12.1.

Although useful in the medical field, medical terminology has a way of dismantling the client–counselor relationship by making the counselor assume the expert role.

Avoid	Use instead
• Sodium	• Salt
• Hyperglycemia	• High blood sugar
• Neuropathy	• Numbness and tingling
• Triglyceride	• Fat in the blood
• Anaphylactic shock	• To stop breathing entirely
• Myocardial infarction	• Heart attack
• Cholecystectomy	• Gallbladder removal

FIGURE 12.1. Examples of medical terms to avoid when speaking with clients.

Use Language That Supports Client Autonomy

In the scenario below, Practitioner A provides an example of what not to do. In the scenario, the practitioner is talking to an insulin-dependent diabetic who is hospitalized after accidently taking too much insulin. The practitioner has seen the client for outpatient diabetes education prior to the incident, but the client is still figuring out how to best manage her blood sugars.

"I know you know this stuff. We've gone over this. You know you must test your blood sugar before meals. Then you have to count the number of carbohydrates you're about to eat and give yourself the correct amount of insulin. Each 15-gram serving requires 1 unit of insulin coverage. If you continue on this path I'm afraid you're going to kill yourself."

By using such confrontational language, the practitioner risks making the client feel ashamed for not dosing her insulin properly. By using the terms "you must" and "you have to" the practitioner essentially removes client autonomy entirely. Saying, "I know you know this stuff" makes the client feel put down, as if she intentionally disappointed her counselor. To finish it off, the counselor uses highly inflammatory rhetoric intended to scare the client into compliance. This type of scare tactic can easily backfire, leaving the client feeling hopeless and unmotivated. Alternatively, Practitioner B uses language that supports client autonomy.

"If it's OK with you, we can review your insulin treatment plan and see if something needs to be adjusted. You're on a carbohydrate-counting insulin treatment plan, which works by using two types of insulin. Ten units of Lantus is given each night and Humalog is injected before eating carbohydrates. The dose of Humalog depends on the number of grams of carbohydrates you plan to eat. This type of insulin works best if 1 unit is injected for each 15-gram serving of carbohydrates eaten. If taken incorrectly, too much insulin causes the type of black-out episode you had yesterday."

In the second scenario, the practitioner provides the information as objectively as possible, after asking permission. She leaves out "you must" and "you are supposed to." In fact, she omits the word "you" altogether. By using such neutral language, the client is left to decide what she'll do from here.

Elicit

Finish an information exchange by asking the client what she thinks or how she feels about the information. Here are some examples of a final elicit:

"What do you think?"
"What do you make of all this?"
"I wonder what your reaction is to this."
"How would that work for you?"
"What else would you like to know about how this works?"

You can also reflect the client's nonverbal cues as a way to elicit a response.

"You look confused. What can I make clearer?"
"This information seems to have upset you. What part do you disagree with?"
"That seems to have resonated with you. Which part did you like?"

E-P-E is a useful tool when attempting to correct misinformation because it allows the practitioner to assess the client's understanding before providing information, while at the same time promoting consistent inter-action and engagement. A summary of the E-P-E technique for correcting misinformation is provided in Figure 12.2.

Clarifying misinformation requires the practitioner to provide infor-mation contrary to what the client already thinks or believes is correct. In order to provide this information in a respectful way the practitioner uses the same principles of information exchange with new information. Elicit the client's understanding of the information, gauge interest in having the information corrected, and ask permission to provide it. Then proceed with presenting the information using language that supports autonomy and avoids information overload. Close your presentation by eliciting the client's response with true curiosity for her perspective and its potential effect on her decision moving forward. Misinformation not only comes

---

Elicit
- Assess for information gaps, gauge interest, or ask permission.
- "What foods strike you as being particularly high in sugar?"
- "What would you like to talk about today? We could review foods high in carbohydrates, your target blood sugar ranges, symptoms of high and low blood sugar, or another topic."
- "If it's OK with you, we could go over this handout I have of foods that raise your blood sugars."

Provide
- Provide brief information snippets.
- Gauge interest level and understanding by looking at changes in nonverbal cues while you talk.
- Avoid jargon and use common terms instead.
  ◊ *Salt* instead of *sodium*.
  ◊ *High blood sugar* instead of *hyperglycemia*.
- If you feel it necessary to explain metabolic processes, do so with simple analogies.

Elicit
- Check in for understanding, engagement, and interest level.
- "What do you make of this?"
- "What's your reaction to this?"
- "What do you think?"

FIGURE 12.2. E-P-E to clarify misinformation.

from external sources, but also from internal sources. These internal or "core" beliefs have the same effect on behavior as simple misinformation but require a little more work to evoke and discuss.

EXPLORING UNHEALTHY BELIEFS ABOUT FOOD, BODY IMAGE, AND EXERCISE

Internal misinformation refers to that which your clients tell themselves about food, exercise, and their bodies. This type of information may or may not have come from another resource. It may even be a compilation of many sources. Detecting unhealthy beliefs, or those based on incorrect information, is an important focus within MI. Within the nutrition and fitness professions, a primary goal is to help clients improve their relationship with food and discover enjoyable

Unhealthy beliefs about nutrition and exercise can negatively influence emotional and social health, thereby hurting one's overall health and well-being.

ways to move their bodies. Dietary and activity patterns are important, but physical health is only one dimension of health. Unhealthy beliefs about nutrition and exercise can negatively influence emotional and social health, thereby hurting one's overall health and well-being.

The spirit of MI is ideal for exploring unhealthy beliefs. You will notice a client's belief system seems to slowly permeate the room as you start to engage, evoke, and reflect what you hear. Resist the righting reflex and focus on evoking those beliefs while expressing compassion, empathy, and self-worth whether or not you agree with them.

By asking open-ended questions about the client's previous experiences with health counselors, diets, and exercise programs, the client provides small morsels of information that give you an idea about her attitude on certain topics. A simple statement such as "I don't bring ice cream into the house" highlights an important theme within the client's belief system about food and her locus of control. Listen for statements that expose the client's attitudes as you go along. Consider the following dialogue and the beliefs the client alludes to. The practitioner uses complex reflections and open-ended questions to engage and evoke more from the client. Once the client and practitioner unpack the origins of the thought or feeling, they can begin exploring whether there is truth in the belief and how the internal misinformation may have kept the client from making a positive health change in the past.

> CLIENT: I don't bring ice cream into the house. That way I'm not tempted.
>
> PRACTITIONER: You believe you cannot be trusted with a whole container of ice cream. You think you'll lose control. [continuing the paragraph reflection]
>
> CLIENT: I don't think I will. I know I will.
>
> PRACTITIONER: At what age do you remember first thinking that you couldn't be trusted with food? [closed-ended question]
>
> CLIENT: Oh, gosh . . . probably 9 or 10.
>
> PRACTITIONER: What happened to make you think that you couldn't control yourself around food? [open-ended question—evoking]
>
> CLIENT: I remember it exactly, actually. I was spending the summer with my grandparents. It was after dinner one night. I think I may even have gone to bed already, but I still wanted something to eat. I crept out to the kitchen to get a snack and my grandma found me poking through the refrigerator. She said to me, "Why can't you just stop eating?" I can feel my stomach tense now the way it did then. I didn't have an answer for her. I still don't know why I can't stop eating.

PRACTITIONER: When your grandmother said, "Why can't you just stop eating?" what you really heard was, "There is something wrong with you." You've held that belief for some time now. [reflection]

This example comes from a chronic dieter who has lived her whole life under the assumption that there was something wrong with her and she could not be trusted with food. Other beliefs common among chronic dieters are:

"I won't get enough to eat."
"I don't deserve to eat what my body wants."
"I won't be able to handle my negative emotions without food."
"Food is the enemy."

Changing these core beliefs starts with identifying them and reflecting them back to the client in a clear and concise way. Allow the client to consider the statement objectively. Is it true? It may have made sense at one point in time, but is it true in the present moment? In discussing unhealthy beliefs about food, fitness, and body image, practitioners often draw upon principles from cognitive-behavioral therapy (CBT), a treatment strategy that focuses on changing thought patterns as a gateway to changing feelings and, ultimately, client actions (Beck, 2005). More on CBT is discussed in Chapter 14. In the dialogue below, the practitioner marries MI and CBT to address internal misinformation and evoke change talk for taking steps to improve body image. The practitioner in the script below senses an unhealthy belief may be at the core of the client's distaste for clothes shopping. She engages and evokes with reflections and open-ended questions. The practitioner asks permission before offering solutions.

CLIENT: Ugh, I hate shopping. I only go if I absolutely have to, and then it's in and out. I don't even try things on anymore. If it doesn't work out, I'll just take it back later.

PRACTITIONER: Shopping is a rather arduous experience for you. [reflection] What is it about shopping that turns you off so much? [open-ended question]

CLIENT: It's just hard to shop when you're at this size. Nothing fits right. I always have to dig through all the normal sizes, and even then I might not find my size. I am just so tired of this. Going into the dressing room and coming out with nothing is too much.

PRACTITIONER: You feel defeated when nothing fits. [reflection]

CLIENT: That's a good word for it. I do feel defeated. I just don't have the energy for it anymore.

PRACTITIONER: It's exhausting to constantly be let down and disappointed when you go shopping. [reflection] I wonder if talking about ways to improve your body image might be a good focus for us today. [asking permission] It's just one thing we could talk about; what else might you want to talk about today? [focusing]

CLIENT: I have hated my body for a long time. I see other overweight women embracing their bodies, but I just don't know how they can do it. They seem happier, though.

PRACTITIONER: You'd like to be happier in your own skin too. [reflection]

CLIENT: I *would* like to be happier in my own skin. [change talk]

PRACTITIONER: It would make you feel better about yourself if you were able to accept your body as it is today. [reflecting change talk]

These are pretty disturbing thought patterns that are common among clients hoping to lose weight. Although common, they are destructive to self-esteem, often fuel overeating, and sabotage efforts at reconstructing a healthy relationship with food. Drawing attention to this negative inner dialogue is the first step in helping clients change it.

PRACTITIONER: How would quieting your inner self-critic improve your life? [open-ended question]

CLIENT: I'd probably go out more often and I'd definitely enjoy shopping more. [change talk]

PRACTITIONER: You're noticing some real benefits to improving your body image. Your inner dialogue is making it miserable for you. [brief summary] What do you think about trying an experiment to help neutralize that voice and make it a little easier to shop? [asking permission]

CLIENT: What are you thinking?

PRACTITIONER: I'm thinking that the shopping itself is not painful, but your thought patterns are. If you work on changing those, dressing yourself in clothes that flatter and fit you can be a way of treating yourself with respect instead of making you miserable. People don't usually change when they feel bullied and put down, even by themselves. They change because they feel inspired and supported. Right now, you seem to be your own bully. [provide] What do you think? [elicit]

CLIENT: But how can I change that? It only seems to get worse as I get older.

PRACTITIONER: That's where the experiment comes in. During the next week, when you find yourself feeling low or defeated, you could pay attention to the inner voice and what it's saying to you. Some clients even find it's useful to grab a scrap of paper and write down everything it says in exactly the words it uses. By shining a light on all the hateful things you say to yourself, you bring it out of the shadows and take away its power. [provide] How do you feel about that idea? [elicit]

CLIENT: Yeah, I see what you're saying.

PRACTITIONER: If you'd like, you can bring your paper back here next week and we can go over it together. [provide]

CLIENT: It sounds hard. There's a lot in there that I'm not sure I want to fess up to, but I need to do something if I want to get better. [change talk]

PRACTITIONER: It sounds scary, but you're up for the challenge and see how conquering this fear could radically improve your life. [reflection of change talk plus affirmation]

This entire dialogue came about by the practitioner picking up on the underlying belief that the client felt she was abnormal and would never reach her goals. CBT exercises that highlight negative self-talk are powerful tools within topics on body image. In nutrition and fitness counseling it all tends to be connected. One's relationship with food, exercise, and body image can be a microcosm of how one functions in the world. Chronic dieters, for example, operate under the assumption that they do not deserve to eat when they are hungry; they think they are insatiable creatures that require external forces to restrict their eating behaviors and protect them from themselves. Evoking these core beliefs about self-worth and the basic rights to feel nourished and whole must sometimes be addressed before meaningful change can occur.

> *Evoking these core beliefs about self-worth and the basic rights to feel nourished and whole must sometimes be addressed before meaningful change can occur.*

Whether destructive health beliefs arise from a pervasive culture that tells people that eating chocolate is indulgent and sinful or from caregivers who imply that children can't trust their own hunger and fullness cues, misinformation clouds and confounds clients' attempts to engage in changes that positively affect health and well-being. Knowing how to evoke and address external and internal misinformation can deepen engagement and foster an environment where clients feel free to discuss the issues that actually have an effect on change.

PART V

A Closer Look at Motivational Interviewing in Nutrition and Fitness Industries

CHAPTER 13

Putting Motivational Interviewing to Work in Nutrition Counseling

There are no good or bad foods. Just foods I love and those I don't.
—MICHELLE MAY

You may be a font of nutrition knowledge, but the key to nutrition counseling isn't just what you know about food and the human body; it's also what you know about your client. Dietary changes can be challenging, as many clients have emotional and cultural ties to food. Solutions to everyday eating dilemmas are often individualized. No one meal plan can promise optimal health for everyone, just as no single routine can help one to quit smoking or improve sleep habits.

Nutrition recommendations are better received when offered within the context of a client's experiences. In the spirit of MI, the client is the expert, knowing exactly which nutritional changes are feasible. Your client doesn't need you to be the food police. What she needs is a practitioner who is interested in coming alongside and supporting her in managing her disease or condition as she discovers which foods make her feel alive, energetic, satisfied, and give a sense of well-being.

The purpose of this chapter is to connect the dots between MI and topics commonly encountered in nutrition and dietetics. Many topics arise in nutrition counseling, such as adding more fruits and vegetables, reducing sugar-sweetened beverages, or emotional eating. While it's impossible to address all topics that may arise in nutrition counseling, in this chapter we highlight a few key topics that commonly surface during nutrition appointments, including dietary changes to manage disease, meal planning, increasing dietary variety, and coping with food cravings that result in overeating.

DIETARY CHANGES NECESSARY FOR DISEASE MANAGEMENT

A new diagnosis that requires dietary management can overwhelm some clients. They often arrive at the office of a nutrition practitioner looking for lists of foods they can eat and foods they will need to avoid. They are hungry for meal ideas and often overwhelmed with concern for managing their disease and required medications. Some are frightened and ready for action and others are angry and hesitant to consider change.

The engaging process of a motivational interviewing session provides the perfect opportunity to ask the client about the new diagnosis. Questions might include:

"What was it like to receive that diagnosis?"
"What concerns you most about the diagnosis?"
"How might this diagnosis change the way you do things?"

The client may not be ready for information. At first, he may just need a sounding board, someone to listen and to empathize. The overwhelming nature of new diagnoses provides opportunities to demonstrate compassion.

New diagnoses will not only affect dietary needs, but may also influence medication regimens and a need for other lifestyle changes such as smoking cessation or stress management. Therefore, dietary changes may take a back seat to more pressing lifestyle changes. In using MI, the practitioner can encourage the client to focus on the changes that are most important to the client, accepting that at times this may not be nutrition.

It's important not to overwhelm the client with facts, figures, and food rules.

For the client who is ready to make dietary changes, consider the speed of change. In some cases, the client may need to make dramatic changes right away. For example, a client diagnosed with lactose intolerance may choose to make an immediate reduction in lactose that will alleviate symptoms. In other cases, the client may choose to make small, gradual changes. Making small changes over time will likely increase the client's self-efficacy and result in lasting change. For example, a client diagnosed with heart disease may begin by replacing high-fat meats for leaner choices, changing from whole milk to 2%, or from cooking with butter to cooking with olive oil. Each small change that is successfully made builds the client's confidence for attempting the next change.

It's important not to overwhelm the client with facts, figures, and food rules. Take the time to set the course and collaborate on what topics to discuss. By focusing with the client, you give him or her the autonomy to decide what you'll talk about. Miller and Rollnick's agenda-mapping technique from Chapter 3 can help to focus the conversation faster. Use menu options to describe changes your clients typically make with these conditions and allow the client to find a starting place that feels manageable. A dietitian might say the following:

> "I have a list here of changes that clients with diabetes often make. May I show it to you? ["Yes."] Here you will see some ideas like adding physical activity, spacing meals or snacks more frequently throughout the day, adding fiber and protein to meals and snacks, and reducing sugar sweetened beverages. Which, if any, from this list sound like a good place to start?"

For clients who are ready to make changes to food choices and eating patterns, recommended dietary modifications can provide opportunities for expanding their meal repertoire. While clients may see a necessary dietary change as negative, it can be reframed as an opportunity to experience new flavors and textures in the kitchen. For example, a client with a new diagnosis of celiac disease will be encouraged to switch from flour tortillas to corn tortillas to eliminate gluten. The client may discover that she enjoys quesadillas made out of corn tortillas more than flour tortillas. She may begin to try new recipes and foods that she might never have discovered had it not been for her new diagnosis.

Many patients diagnosed with diseases are able to see the blessing in disguise; they often say that they appreciate the newfound motivation for eating well. An individual with diabetes may discover that, thanks to the dietary and exercise changes that were necessary for managing his blood sugars, he now has more energy. Clients will also appreciate hearing that taste buds change over time. Therefore, a reduction in table salt may make the food taste bland at first. However, in just a few weeks, the client may discover a new enjoyable flavor that was previously masked by the salt.

Helping clients discover the silver lining of diet-based changes can reduce perceived barriers. However, when discussing these topics it's easy to fall into the cheerleading trap. Within an MI session, these tips and tricks are provided gently and with a tone of empathy and autonomy, as in the following scenario:

> "Many of my clients, like you, are less than enthused about switching from whole milk to skim milk. There is certainly a significant difference in taste. Can I share some tips that other clients have found useful? ["Yes."] First, clients find this change easier to make in a gradual step-down fashion. They usually start by mixing whole milk and 2% for a few days, and then drink only 2%. Once they are accustomed to that, then they start mixing 2% and 1% and eventually switch to 1%, then mix 1% with skim, and eventually drink mainly skim milk. Also

they find that their taste buds adapt, and what at first seemed watery and bland becomes enjoyable. What do you make of this information? What do you think would work best for you?"

If the practitioner can guide the client toward small, manageable changes that maximize taste and minimize preparation time, the client will be more likely to stick with the change. At times, dietary changes require significant adjustments in meal planning and cooking techniques. With the help of an MI practitioner, these dietary adjustments can be made gradually, in accordance with the client's readiness to change. Often, even the most subtle dietary change results in a need to make adjustments in meal planning and preparation.

MEAL PREPARATION AND PLANNING

Many of us attempt to manage full lives complete with work and family. We cram in as many activities as our lives will hold until our schedules are busting at the seams. We aim for more home-cooked, sit-down meals, but the barriers to achieving this goal are often immense. Many turn to the convenience of restaurants and packaged meals when in a pinch. While eating out can provide a break from the cooking and cleaning, frequent stops for takeout can be costly and can lead to overeating. Furthermore, it can be especially challenging to find a variety of options that meet the nutritional needs of your clients who may have necessary dietary restrictions for managing disease.

Most dietary changes require a tweak in meal preparation, meal planning, or both. Ultimately, a client's ability to manage such changes depends on contextual skills. Child feeding expert and registered dietitian Ellyn Satter (2008) defines contextual skills as "skills and resources for managing the food context and orchestrating family meals" (p. 225). Developing strong contextual skills is about gaining the skills to prepare regular and reliable meals and snacks and eating those at times that honor internal hunger cues.

Where is your client getting stuck when it comes to planning for eating?

Where is your client getting stuck when it comes to planning for eating? Is it that she hardly knows how to boil water and lacks confidence in the kitchen? Or does she perceive cooking as something that requires a long, labor-intensive process? Is she paralyzed with fear because she worries that her meals don't always include a perfect mix of all the essential vitamins and minerals? Perhaps she hasn't found a grocery-shopping schedule that easily fits into her busy week. Before any planning or goal setting can occur, it's useful to explore her concerns. What are her barriers to meal planning and preparation? Only then can you provide her with the support she needs to be successful both at the grocery store and in the kitchen.

The Grocery Store: Planning for Eating

Once your client expresses interest in making changes to her meal planning strategies, it's important to first assess her current skills and patterns. How often does she like to go to the grocery store? How does she decide which foods to purchase? Does she go with specific meals in mind, make up meal ideas while wandering the grocery store aisles, or does she buy random items and then later attempt to turn those items into meals? Specific evoking questions can be used to invite the client to explore which pieces of her current meal-planning strategy are working and which pieces are not. Here are some open-ended questions that may help her along in the process:

> "Describe your current grocery-shopping system. How do you determine what you will eat for the week?"
> "What's working well for you in how you plan your meals?"
> "What's not working well for you in how you plan your meals?"
> "Which part, if any, of the way you plan your meals are you interested in changing?"
> "How do you see this change improving other areas of your life?"
> "What resources would you need to be successful if you were to make this change in the way you plan your meals?"

These questions will help the client to home in on the real issue. In true MI fashion, when the client seems ready, invite her to devise solutions to her stumbling blocks. You are there to provide suggestions *only* if she gets stuck. We each have meal-planning strategies that work for us; however, these same strategies may not work for your client. In the script below, the practitioner puts the client in the driver's seat to determine what might work best. The practitioner also helps the client when she gets stuck.

> PRACTITIONER: You mentioned that you'd like to eat out less often. [reflection] What time of the day or which meals did you have in mind? [open-ended question]
>
> CLIENT: Definitely dinner. My boyfriend and I eat dinner out about four times a week. It was fun when we were first dating, but we've each put on a few pounds in the last 6 months, and we're trying to save up money to go on vacation. [change talk—desire for change]

PRACTITIONER: You've noticed the cost savings of preparing more meals at home. [reflection]

CLIENT: Yes. Some nights, between the appetizer, drinks, and meal, we spend as much as $50 between the two of us.

PRACTITIONER: You're finding that it adds up quickly. [reflection]

CLIENT: It really does.

PRACTITIONER: What would need to change in order for you to prepare more meals at home? [open-ended question]

CLIENT: We would need to get to the grocery store more often and maybe have more of a plan when we go. Sometimes we say, "Oh, let's stay home tonight and just fix something." And then we open up our cupboards and can't find anything to make, so we head out.

PRACTITIONER: You'd really like a fully stocked kitchen so that you're less tempted to eat out. [reflection]

CLIENT: Yes. I mean, we both know how to make a few things, so that's not the issue. It's just that we need to do a better job at the grocery store. [change talk—the need to change]

PRACTITIONER: You've got the cooking part down; you just want help on the meal planning and the grocery shopping. That's where you see things could change for the better. [reflection of change talk] What ideas do you have? [open-ended question]

CLIENT: I think I just need to make sure I make a list or something before I go. [change talk—activation]

PRACTITIONER: Yes, a list is something that works for some people. You want to be more organized when you go to the store. You want to have a plan. Would you be interested in hearing a few shopping list strategies that my other clients have tried? [asking permission]

CLIENT: Sure!

PRACTITIONER: One idea is to write out a grocery list that includes food for a certain number of dinner meals each week . . . maybe four or five. Then go to the grocery store with both your list of ingredients and the meals you plan to make for dinner written down. Some clients prefer to go to the grocery store every 3 days or so, while others prefer once a week. Some like to buy major nonperishable items, like canned beans and canned tomato sauce, once a month and then only buy the fresh produce, dairy, and meat items once a week. [giving information] Which, if any, of these sounds more like you? [open-ended question]

CLIENT: I really don't like going to the grocery store very often, so I could see how planning out my meals and only going once a week would probably work best.

PRACTITIONER: You'd like to change the way you've been doing things by being more organized and including meal ideas on your list before heading to the store. [reflection] Which days are best for grocery shopping each week? [open-ended question]

CLIENT: I like going Friday nights because it's quiet, so probably just on the way home from work.

PRACTITIONER: OK, Friday nights. [reflection] If you were to do your grocery shopping on Friday nights, when would be the best time to write up your list? [open-ended question]

CLIENT: Probably Thursday night before I go to bed. Then I can just put the list in my purse and have it with me when I drive home from work on Fridays.

PRACTITIONER: All right, so what you're thinking is if you can spend a few minutes coming up with certain meal ideas and writing those down Thursday nights, then it will be easy for you to shop Fridays on your way home from work. [summary] How will your boyfriend feel about this change and how can he support you? [open-ended question]

CLIENT: He'll totally be on board with this. I think it might even be fun at first to test out our cooking skills. He can support me by giving me ideas for meals we can make together.

PRACTITIONER: You and your boyfriend seem excited about planning more meals to cook at home each week. [reflection] What sort of goal would you like to set in terms of the number of dinners you eat out each week? [open-ended question]

CLIENT: I think if we could go from eating four meals out each week to eating one meal out each week that would be great.

PRACTITIONER: You'd like to shoot for eating out only one day a week. How confident are you on a scale from 0 to 10 that you can reach this goal, with 10 being very confident and 0 being not at all confident?

In this conversation the practitioner uses consistent reflective listening to evoke and reinforce change talk. She also invites the client to take the lead in figuring out the pieces of the puzzle. The practitioner asks the client how and when, provides some information, but gives the client autonomy in deciding what might work best for her. She ends by summarizing the specific goal the client has set and exploring confidence and any potential barriers that may arise as the client attempts this change.

In the Kitchen: Preparing Meals

If your client expresses interest in expanding his repertoire of meals and snacks prepared at home, it's important first to determine his baseline cooking skills and build from there. What does he already know how to make? What does he make regularly? What other foods, if any, would he like to be able to make? How much time does he prefer to spend in the kitchen preparing meals? Snacks? While assessing the client's contextual skills in the kitchen, it's easy to fall victim to the question–answer trap. As you gather this information, use open-ended questions that allow the client to tell his story.

> "Tell me about the foods you eat on a regular basis."
> "What would you commonly eat for dinner?"
> "What are your go-to meals?"
> "What kinds of foods do you reach for when you're in a rush?"
> "If you can remember, tell me what you had for breakfasts this past week."
> "What other foods, if any, would you like to be able to make?"

You can help increase your client's self-efficacy for cooking by giving him quick and easy meal ideas, if needed. He may not realize that a balanced meal can be made in as little as 10 to 15 minutes. Handout 13.1 includes examples of meals that require minimal time and basic cooking skills.

There are many resources available for expanding one's meal ideas. We all get into cooking ruts and crave new and exciting food experiences. Nutrition counselors can provide tangible food ideas for clients within an MI session. The key is simply asking permission before providing these ideas and offering resources that best meet your clients' needs.

In order to provide relevant meal ideas, first assess your client's preferred tastes and textures. In addition, consider that many clients have cultural food preferences that are important to understand. A common mistake of nutrition counselors is to start spouting off meal and recipe ideas without checking in with the client first to determine food preferences. By asking these first, the client will feel respected and understood.

Before providing new meal ideas, determine your client's cooking skills. Recipes have very limited information to guide an actual cooking event. Encourage your client with limited cooking skills to start with very basic and simple endeavors. When discussing different recipes, assess the client's interest in the recipe and perceived ability to prepare the recipe by asking open-ended questions. A scaling question may also be useful, such

FRUITS AND VEGETABLES MADE EASY

10 Meals in 15 Minutes

Are you hungry, but short on time? Here are 10 quick, easy meal ideas that include fruits and vegetables, along with a shopping list to take with you the next time you head for the grocery store.

1. **Hummus Wrap**
   Tortilla, fresh spinach, hummus, slice of cheese
2. **Chili Baked Potato**
   Potato, canned chili (there are vegetarian options), shredded cheese
3. **Pita Pizza**
   Pita bread, pesto or pizza sauce, mozzarella cheese, toppings such as bell pepper, olives, mushrooms, and Canadian bacon
4. **Cottage Cheese or Yogurt, Fruit, and Granola**
   Cottage cheese or yogurt, fruit, granola
5. **Grilled Cheese and Tomato or Vegetable Soup**
   Bread, cheese, favorite soup
6. **Breakfast Burrito**
   Tortilla, scrambled eggs, salsa, canned black beans, shredded cheese
7. **Taco Bowl**
   Canned beans, instant rice, canned or frozen corn, shredded cheese, tomatoes, avocado, salsa
8. **Tomato Tuna Melt**
   Bread, bagel, or English muffin, sliced tomato, tuna with mayonnaise, cheese
9. **Peanut Butter and Banana on Bread or Tortilla**
   Bread or tortilla, peanut butter, banana
10. **Lettuce-Free Salad**
    Canned beans of your choice (garbanzo beans work well), small vegetables such as peas and baby tomatoes, diced vegetables such as bell pepper, cucumber, and carrots, vinaigrette salad dressing of your choice

---

GROCERY LIST

Produce	Canned	Refrigerated	Grain	Misc
Fresh spinach	Chili	Shredded mozzarella	Pita bread	Peanut butter
Bell pepper	Tuna	Slices of provolone,	Tortillas	Mayonnaise
Mushrooms	Black beans (2)	jack or cheddar	Bread, bagel or	Salad dressing
Fruit of your	Garbonzo beans	Hummus	English muffin	Salsa
choice	Tomato or	Pesto	Instant rice	
Avocado	vegetable soup	Eggs	Granola	
Tomato	Corn	Canadian bacon		
Cucumber		Cottage cheese or		
Carrots		yogurt		

(continued)

15 Ways to Sneak Fruits and Vegetables into Your Meals and Snacks

Everyone knows the power of produce. Food fads have come and gone, but fruits and vegetables have held steady at the top of recommended food lists. They are colorful, tasty, versatile, and full of vitamins, minerals and fiber; yet they're easily overlooked at the grocery store. Here are just a few ways fruits and vegetables can liven up even the most boring dish.

1. Fruit smoothies or juicing
2. Baked potato with vegetable toppings such as beans, salsa, and broccoli
3. Precut vegetables dipped in salad dressing or hummus
4. Apple, banana, or celery with peanut butter or other nut butter
5. Soups with vegetables and/or legumes
6. One-pot entrees with vegetables included such as casseroles, stir fries, pasta, and stews
7. A lettuce- or spinach-based side salad
8. A lettuce- or spinach-based main salad with added chicken, tuna, salmon, bacon, steak, or beans
9. A lettuce-free salad side dish (salad toppings only, mixed with salad dressing)
10. Fresh vegetable such as broccoli or cauliflower, steamed in the microwave, flavored with cheese, butter, salt, and/or other seasonings
11. Add vegetables such as lettuce, tomatoes, avocado, and corn to a burrito, taco, or taco salad
12. Add vegetables to entrees such as sandwiches, wraps, pizza, and omelets
13. Add salsa to anything
14. Add frozen spinach to scrambled eggs, omelets, or quiches
15. Add vegetables into a pasta, rice, or quinoa salad

as, "How likely are you to prepare this recipe on a scale from 0 to 10, with 0 being not at all likely and 10 being very likely?"

Determine your client's preference for obtaining recipes. Does he like using the Internet? Apps? Cookbooks? Or does he prefer to ask a trusted friend? For a client who is faced with a challenge of reducing dietary sodium, the practitioner may offer strategies for replacing table salt with other seasonings, or refer the client to a website or cookbook with low-sodium meal ideas. It all depends on your client's preference.

Finally, ask the client how long he prefers to spend preparing and cleaning up from meals. Recommend recipe ideas that line up with his availability. For clients who have limited time, consider suggesting one-pot meals to minimize dishes and mixing premade items with fresh items to save time on preparation. For example, jarred spaghetti sauce may be an important time saver for some clients. Others may rely on prechopped, frozen, or canned vegetables and canned beans. Keeping recipes simple is key in increasing self-efficacy in the kitchen. Clients will be more open to trying new meal ideas if their preferences for taste, texture, and cooking techniques are determined first. Figure 13.1 includes a list of topics that are useful to explore with the client before providing recipe tips and suggestions.

Here are some additional questions that can be used to assess your client's needs for guidance in the kitchen.

"How comfortable are you in the kitchen?"

"How long do you prefer to spend preparing a (breakfast, lunch, dinner) meal?"

"Describe your preferred cooking methods. (Do you prefer baking, boiling, sautéing, microwaving, grilling, etc.?)"

"What are your preferences in terms of taste, texture, and ethnic cuisine?"

Before providing suggestions for new meals ideas, determine your client's:
- Current preferences of tastes and textures.
- Current staple meals.
- Cultural food preferences.
- Preferred time spent in the kitchen.
- Preferred method for finding new recipes.
- Necessary dietary restrictions based on disease state or condition and medications.
- Cooking skills.
- Budget for food.

FIGURE 13.1. Ask before you provide.

"Describe the meals you know how to make and enjoy making."
"What flavors, textures, colors, or food groups are you hoping to add to your meals?"
"How do you prefer to obtain new recipes or meal ideas?"

In the script below the practitioner asks some of these questions and guides the client toward a behavior change that the she perceives as manageable.

PRACTITIONER: You've set your own goal of limiting your eating out to once a week. You've figured out a grocery-shopping strategy that involves going on Friday evenings with a list. [summary] Now I'm wondering if it would be helpful to talk about *what* you're going to cook. Would you be interested in discussing this piece further? [focusing and asking permission]

CLIENT: Yes, that would be helpful. Like I said, I have a few meals that I know how to make, but I know if I expanded that list, I'd be more excited to cook at home [change talk—reasons for change]. When I've tried in the past to cook at home more, I always felt like I was eating the same foods over and over again.

PRACTITIONER: Eating a variety is important to you. [affirmation]

CLIENT: Yes. And since I work, I don't have a lot of time to create these elaborate meals.

PRACTITIONER: So taste is important; you mentioned earlier that cost is important, and it sounds like time matters too. [summary] What else is important to you as we figure out the best meals for cooking at home? [open-ended question]

CLIENT: I love Italian and Mexican food, and of course American comfort foods are good too. I don't know how to make Chinese food, but I like it.

PRACTITIONER: Great, many cuisines to choose from. [reflection] First tell me about the foods you already make. [open-ended question]

CLIENT: I make good spaghetti. I've made that for my boyfriend and he loves it. I also make a pesto ravioli dish where you just buy the prepared ravioli and the container of pesto and put it together. I'll sometimes add whatever vegetables I have on hand to that. Let's see . . . if I'm feeling lazy, I'll make a quesadilla in the microwave. I've found those precooked chicken breasts at the store and will sometimes add those to whatever I'm cooking. That's about it. Maybe a few others, but not very many.

PRACTITIONER: OK, those are some good ones. You already have some great ideas about putting convenient, time-saving foods together to make an overall healthy and tasty meal. [affirmation] If it's OK with you let's also talk about how you can branch out and try some new and exciting dishes. [asking permission] How do you prefer to find recipes? [open-ended question] Do you like using the Internet? Cookbooks? Or do you like to watch cooking shows? [closed-ended probing questions]

CLIENT: Oh yes, all of those methods work.

PRACTITIONER: The Internet is a great resource for free recipes. And sometimes just browsing the recipes in the "Quick and Easy" recipe collection can get those creative juices flowing. [giving information] I can give you some of my clients' favorite recipe websites, if you'd like? I also have some quick, easy recipe ideas here on this handout [Handout 13.1]. Would you be interested in taking a look at this together? [giving a menu of options and asking permission]

CLIENT: Yes, that would be great.

PRACTITIONER: As you glance at this handout, which, if any of these sounds like something you'd like to try? [open-ended question]

EXPANDING FOOD VARIETY

Variety is not only the spice of life, but instrumental in ensuring a diet full of essential vitamins and minerals. Children and adults often have very limited food acceptance. The term *food acceptance* is defined by Ellyn Satter (2008) as being comfortable with the foods you like, flexible about the foods you choose, and interested in new foods, discovering ways to learn to like them. Picky-eating children often grow up into finicky adults with nutritional deficits that can contribute to chronic disease. Many adults have limited food acceptance, and we do our best to cater to their needs when we invite them to dinner. However, what if the picky eater is your client?

If your client has a limited food selection and is interested in trying new foods and expanding his variety, invite him to brainstorm a list of foods preferred, foods detested, and foods in between (neither liked nor hated). Ask open-ended questions to determine the origin of the food dislikes. It can be useful to assess whether the repulsion is due to flavor, texture, appearance, or a traumatic childhood event. If he's interested, explain that it often requires several exposures to a new food before it is accepted. Invite him to select a food from either the foods detested or the foods in between list and begin discussing how he would go about preparing this food, if he were to try it again.

With permission, invite him to consider trying that novel food with a food that he likes. For example, if he dislikes cauliflower but likes cheese, perhaps he'd be more willing to try the cauliflower if it's smothered in cheese. Toppings such as cheeses, sauces, salad dressings, and butter can dramatically improve the taste of a disliked food. Many refrain from using these items out of concern for nutrition. However, these items may be necessary at first to increase palatability. Over time, the client will likely find that large amounts of the topping may not be necessary for long-term enjoyment. And for clients who require a dietary restriction to manage a disease or condition, nutritionally altered products can be used. For example, if ranch dressing is helpful for increasing acceptance of bell peppers, and the client is concerned about dietary fat, then a low-fat ranch dressing can be used.

Many fail to meet the recommended dietary guidelines for fruits and vegetables. Therefore, assisting a client in expanding his food variety often means exposing him to new fruits and vegetables. Clients who eat inadequate amounts of these foods often voice a number of barriers including taste, the perishable nature of fresh produce, cost, and a general lack of skills to prepare them in a pleasurable way. Clients can use a number of strategies to add fruits and vegetables to meals and snacks (Handout 13.1). When providing these ideas, it's important to do so in an E-P-E format. Ideas can be provided in a menu option as in the following script:

> PRACTITIONER: You seem motivated to start adding more fruits and vegetables into your diet. What ideas do you have for how you might go about doing this? [elicit]
>
> CLIENT: I noticed those mandarin oranges are in season right now. I like those because they aren't too messy and easy to take with me. For vegetables, I'm really running out of ideas. I tend to stick to only three different vegetables—corn, carrots, and potatoes.
>
> PRACTITIONER: You're interested in trying some seasonal fruit and feel a bit stuck with your vegetable selection. [reflection] Would you be interested in hearing other ideas? [asking permission] Some of my clients like drinking fruit smoothies for breakfast or adding a banana or berries to cereal in the morning. Others prefer cutting up vegetables ahead of time and enjoying them with lunch or snacks dipped in salad dressing or hummus. Another idea is to add more entrees to your dinner items that have vegetables built in like soups, casseroles, or stir fries. Or perhaps you'd prefer microwaving or steaming fresh, canned, or frozen vegetable side dishes or adding salads. [provide] Which, if any of these ideas would you like to explore further? [elicit]

This is one way to offer suggestions to your client. In the following script, the client reports she has limited acceptance of fruits and vegetables and expresses a desire to expand and try new foods. The practitioner guides her through the planning process by listening for and evoking change talk and reflecting it back, ultimately moving the client through ambivalence and toward change.

> PRACTITIONER: From this list of strategies to reduce constipation, you've selected adding fiber by eating more fruits and vegetables. [reflection] What led you to choose that particular topic? [evoking change talk with an open-ended question]
>
> CLIENT: I know I don't eat enough of them. [change talk—need to change] There aren't very many that I really like. [sustain talk] And I'm sure that eating more would help move things along. [ambivalence]
>
> PRACTITIONER: Despite the fact that you don't care much for fruits and vegetables, you want to challenge yourself in this area and recognize the importance of adding more fruits and vegetables in alleviating your constipation. [reflection of change talk]
>
> CLIENT: Yes. I have a feeling if I just learned how to make fruits and vegetables taste good, I'd probably be able to add more to my diet. [change talk—ability to change]
>
> PRACTITIONER: Preparing fruits and vegetables in a tasty manner sounds like your biggest challenge. [reflection of change talk]
>
> CLIENT: Right.
>
> PRACTITIONER: Can I give you some information about trying new foods that has encouraged other clients?
>
> CLIENT: Yes.
>
> PRACTITIONER: Many of my clients find—and research supports this—that repeatedly trying new foods in different ways increases food acceptance. [giving information] Can you think of a food you used to really despise that now doesn't taste so bad? [closed-ended question]
>
> CLIENT: Oh, that's an easy one—broccoli. I used to hate it. Now it's one of the only vegetables I eat.
>
> PRACTITIONER: Great example. [affirmation] Why do you think your opinion of broccoli changed? [open-ended question]
>
> CLIENT: I don't know. Probably because it came with a few of the dishes I ordered at restaurants and I just kept trying it. This one restaurant I always go to puts butter and lemon juice on it, and it's delicious.
>
> PRACTITIONER: That's a good example of how preparation really can make a difference. And you didn't give up and kept tasting what was on your plate. [affirmation]

CLIENT: Yes, but now I only eat broccoli, carrots, corn, and peas.

PRACTITIONER: OK, so those are the vegetables you prefer. [reflection] What fruits do you like? [open-ended question]

CLIENT: Fruit is easier. I like oranges, grapes, apples, and pineapple. I hate cantaloupe, watermelon, bananas, kiwi, and some berries that are really sour.

PRACTITIONER: Yes, sour fruit or any that isn't quite ripe yet can really ruin the experience of that food. [reflection] Which fruits or vegetables that you don't much care for are you interested in trying again, if any? [open-ended question]

CLIENT: Someone told me about freezing bananas and dipping them in chocolate. I do like chocolate. I could try that.

PRACTITIONER: Great idea. [affirmation] What else?

CLIENT: Oh, tomatoes. I feel like I should give those another try. I'm starting to like salsa, and tomatoes aren't that different from salsa.

PRACTITIONER: Another good idea. [affirmation] What ideas do you have for preparing tomatoes in a way that may be enjoyable? [open-ended question]

CLIENT: I don't know. I mean, I will occasionally try one drowned in salad dressing if it's served at a restaurant.

PRACTITIONER: The salad dressing makes it more palatable. [reflection]

CLIENT: Well, sort of. The mushy center still catches me off guard as it mushes in my mouth.

PRACTITIONER: So it's a texture thing. [reflection]

CLIENT: Yes, but I don't know why salsa doesn't bother me; maybe because it's chopped up.

PRACTITIONER: So perhaps chopping up tomatoes and adding them to your meals might work. What other ideas do you have for adding tomatoes in a way that you won't notice or be turned off by the texture? [open-ended question]

CLIENT: I don't know.

PRACTITIONER: Would you be interested in hearing some ideas? [asking permission]

CLIENT: Yes.

PRACTITIONER: How would you feel about trying to add tomatoes to hot dishes like pastas or soups? [open-ended question, giving information]

CLIENT: Oh yeah, good idea. That could work.

PRACTITIONER: You found two places to start in terms of expanding your fruit and vegetables selection: chocolate-covered bananas and adding tomatoes to soups and pasta. [summary] What additional resources could I provide you to help you with this little eating experiment? [open-ended question]

In this dialogue, the practitioner invites the client to navigate a delicate balance between the discomfort of trying new foods to help manage symptoms (in this case, constipation) while still honoring one's palate. It's important that clients discover foods that both support a healthy body and a pleasurable eating experience. Clients often need significant guidance in discovering and redefining a healthy relationship with food.

COPING WITH CRAVINGS

In an effort to lose weight or manage a disease, many attempt to eliminate certain high-fat, high-sugar, high-calorie foods. Restricting favorite foods might seem easy at first, but then the challenges of life get in the way—a holiday party, a birthday celebration, a tantalizing advertisement for a missed food, or a sad, lonely evening at home with the ice cream container calling from the fridge. For the majority of people, restriction leads to overeating, preoccupation with food, and body dissatisfaction (Polivy et al., 2005; Spoor et al., 2006). Researchers have found that individuals who simply *plan* on dieting will eat more in anticipation of the restriction (Urbszat, Herman, & Polivy, 2002). That's right—just *thinking* about restricting is enough to enhance the urge to eat. In short, restriction is a recipe for overeating.

Habituation

If you were told today that starting tomorrow you would never be able to eat ice cream again, what would you eat tonight? You'd eat ice cream, of course. And chances are good that you'd head to the store to buy a nice big gallon of ice cream even if it was freezing cold outside and the last thing on earth you actually felt like eating. How do you help your clients break this vicious dieting cycle? The answer seems almost counterintuitive, but a growing body of research supports the concept of habituation, or repeated exposure to a stimulus that leads to a decreased response (Epstein, Temple, Roemmich, & Bouton, 2009). In other words, serving the same food over days may result in a decreased desire to eat that food.

At the same time, giving oneself full permission to enjoy satisfying meals and snacks may end the internal battle that plagues dieters. This is because dieters often try to "be good" earlier in the day and then throw in the towel in the evening, scouring the cupboards to satisfy a deprivation that's been building all day. It's the feelings of deprivation paired with guilt that make it hard to tune into internal cues such as hunger, fullness, and cravings, our only internal navigation that tells us what and how much to eat.

Many times, the client's thoughts and worries about food disrupt this internal navigation system. For example, if a client is preoccupied with the fat, carbohydrate, and calories in the chicken Alfredo she's about to eat, she may completely miss that her body is actually craving a salad. The key is turning off the head game and listening to what the body wants and needs. Human beings don't just have cravings for fat, sugar, and salt. Humans are set up to crave the necessary nutrients that are lacking in the diet. Encouraging clients to tune into and trust their internal cues and cravings is a subtle way of supporting client autonomy within the process of change.

Habituation is not about encouraging a client to eat only chocolate until she feels ill and repulsed by it. Instead, it's about supporting your client in giving herself full permission to enjoy chocolate while tuning into how it makes her body feel. Using habituation techniques with previously forbidden foods ultimately alleviates the anxiety of food insecurity for a particular food and thus builds a healthier relationship with that food. Chances are good that your client will crave a variety of foods once the internal food fight has ceased.

Many who struggle with compulsive eating will have a hard time believing they can trust their hunger, fullness, and cravings. Clients will often say, "But I crave chocolate all the time! If I let myself eat it whenever I want it I'll never eat anything else." The client is really saying that she is afraid that she can't be trusted with chocolate. As long as that belief is dominating her thoughts she can be expected to overeat it. But consider guiding the client in exploring her cravings and the belief that's fueling it. Use open-ended questions and reflections to point out the times of the day when she doesn't crave chocolate. For example, she may not crave it first thing in the morning when she's lying in bed. You might even be able to help her realize through a strategic summary that because she doesn't allow herself to enjoy the chocolate while she's eating it, her cravings are actually exacerbated by the feelings of guilt she experiences. If she comes to the realization that something needs to change, you can be there to offer information about the benefits of habituation and suggest an experiment at home.

Chances are good that your client will crave a variety of foods once the internal food fight has ceased.

A little nutrition knowledge can be helpful in guiding the planning of balanced, satisfying meals, but a head full of nutrition rules and regulations could lead to a life of yo-yo dieting. Giving oneself full permission to enjoy favorite foods is a foreign concept and not a message a client expects to receive from her nutritionist. As with any change, baby steps may be necessary to get the client comfortable with enjoying feared foods in moderation.

Mindful Eating

You can also help your clients by teaching them how to slow down the eating experience and to savor preferred foods. Eating mindfully takes practice. Each time your client pauses to check in with her cravings and body signals is a small victory on the path toward developing a healthy relationship with food. It's important to celebrate these little victories by tuning your client into the small successes with affirmations.

How do you introduce mindful eating to clients? Start by having the client talk about her craving. Have her pick one food that she feels most out of control around. Invite her to share how she'd like her relationship to be with that one food. Ask permission before giving information about habituation and mindful eating techniques, and check in to assess her response before moving forward, as in the dialogue below.

PRACTITIONER: You shared that you feel out of control when you have chips and salsa in the house. [reflection] What's that like for you? [open-ended question]

CLIENT: I open up a bag and a jar of salsa and it's game over. I won't stop until the bag is empty.

PRACTITIONER: You eat more than you'd like to eat. [reflection]

CLIENT: Yes, I'd like to eat like my boyfriend—help myself to 10 or 20 chips and move on. [change talk—desire to change]

PRACTITIONER: He doesn't seem preoccupied by the chips. [reflection]

CLIENT: No, it's no big deal to him.

PRACTITIONER: You'd like to no longer feel out of control around chips, more like your boyfriend. [reflection of change talk] Why do you think he's different with chips and salsa? [open-ended question]

CLIENT: I don't know. There really aren't any foods that he's like that with. He doesn't really have to watch his diet. He works construction, so he's always moving around at work and can eat whatever he wants.

PRACTITIONER: You're wondering if the fact that he doesn't diet has something to do with his ability to control himself around chips and salsa. [reflection] You might be on to something. [affirmation] Could I tell you about what the research says regarding dieting and cravings? [asking permission]

CLIENT: Sure.

PRACTITIONER: Researchers are finding that when we tell ourselves we can't or shouldn't eat certain foods, it may actually intensify the craving. Some of my clients find that when they feel guilty after eating the "forbidden" foods, they end up eating more *because* they tell themselves they won't be able to eat it again. [giving information] What do you make of this information? [open-ended question]

CLIENT: Yes, I could see how that might be true. But what am I supposed to do, though? Just eat them all the time?

PRACTITIONER: I'm sure this may sound a little strange, but some of my clients have found that giving themselves permission to eat favorite foods when they crave them results in feeling less out of control in the end. Eating chips and salsa around the clock might get old after a while. I'm sure that's hard to imagine. [giving information] What would your week look like if you left here giving yourself full permission to eat as many chips as you'd like? [open-ended question]

CLIENT: Wow, that sounds a little scary. I'm pretty sure I'd pick some up on my way home and eat them all. [sustain talk]

PRACTITIONER: Yes, that sounds very likely, and it's normal to feel anxious about that. [reflection] What are you typically doing or thinking while you are eating your chips and salsa? [open-ended question]

CLIENT: Sometimes I'm chatting with my boyfriend, or watching TV. I'm not sure.

PRACTITIONER: It sounds like pairing chip-eating with TV and socializing enhances the experience. [reflection]

CLIENT: Yes, in a way, but sometimes I look down at the empty bag and can hardly believe that I ate them all. I don't even realize I'm still eating them sometimes. [implying a desire to change]

PRACTITIONER: You're zoned out for much of the chip-eating experience and it's like you're missing the best part of your day. [complex reflection – picking up on a desire to change]

CLIENT: I know. What's the deal with that?

PRACTITIONER: Would you be willing to try a little experiment? [asking permission]

CLIENT: Yes.

PRACTITIONER: I'm curious what would happen if you gave yourself full permission to eat as many chips and salsa as you wanted from here until our next appointment and if at the same time you slowed down the eating experience and attempted to pay attention to the taste and crunch of the chips and salsa while you are eating. [posing a hypothetical experiment] What do you think might happen? [open-ended question]

CLIENT: I'd probably eat them for a few days, but I can see how I might get tired of them after a while. And I'd probably be really thirsty from all the salt.

PRACTITIONER: You're noticing that your body may not feel so hot on the chips and salsa diet and might start craving other things. [reflection]

As in the dialogue above, take the client through some "what ifs" so that she can envision the eating experience and talk through her fears and reservations of the experiment with someone she trusts. It's also useful to explore the emotional component of eating. It may be that the chips and salsa are helping with a negative emotion. If she were to give herself full permission to eat the chips and remove distractions from her environment to eat mindfully, she may notice negative emotions such as loneliness, sadness, or anxiety start to surface.

As mentioned frequently throughout this book, food and emotions are complex. For a client with binge-eating disorder, extensive therapy by a trained psychotherapist may be needed before a client can conduct a habituation eating exercise like this. (See Appendix 1, "Making Referrals.") It's important to assess your client's history with behaviors such as restriction, binging, purging, and other forms of abuse. Furthermore, some clients may not have the luxury of eating whatever foods they want if dietary manipulation is a necessary therapy in the management or treatment of a disease or condition. For more resources on incorporating non-diet approaches into nutrition counseling sessions, visit Appendix 2, "Additional Resources."

As with all nutritional changes addressed in this chapter, the spirit of MI serves as a guiding force. The following MI strategies are essential in behavior change counseling for dietary change:

- Invite the client to discuss current patterns and motivation for change.
- Reflect and reinforce change talk.
- Ask permission before providing information about change and deliver small bits of information at a time.
- Let the client take the lead in determining which changes she will make and how she will make them.

It's easy for change talk to be cloaked in ambivalence. Clients may want to and know how to change, but need your help in moving through their ambivalence toward change.

CHAPTER 14

Putting Motivational Interviewing to Work in Fitness Counseling

> Don't just add physical activity to your life, add life to your physical activity.
>
> —MICHELLE MAY

The topic of fitness comes up often in health-based counseling. Many people lead sedentary lives, voicing inadequate time and resources for physical activity. For practitioners it may be all too tempting to discard the principles of MI and start giving directions based on the American College of Sports Medicine (ACSM) physical activity guidelines. Just as health professionals do their clients a disservice by directing them to "just eat less," they equally disable them by saying, "just exercise more." This chapter discusses the use of MI when discussing the topics commonly encountered in exercise counseling.

EXPLORING MOTIVATION FOR PHYSICAL ACTIVITY

Like with most behavior changes, motivation for physical activity is complex. Self-determination theory (SDT) brings to light common thoughts and attitudes clients experience when deciding whether or not to be active. SDT is based on the idea that people are naturally self-motivated and eager to succeed because success in and of itself is gratifying and rewarding (Ryan & Deci, 2000). According to the SDT, there are two types of motivation, known commonly as autonomous motivation and controlled motivation.

Autonomous motivation is present when the client finds the activity enjoyable or discovers an immediate positive effect during and directly after exercising. In general, being active aligns with the client's core values and he looks forward to the activity because of the intrinsic benefits and joy of participating. Controlled motivation is the product of internal pressure that a client puts on himself to be physically active as well as any external reward for participating. Clients with controlled motivation may be motivated by competing in a sport to win, tracking activity using an exercise-tracking app or a wrist gadget, and often employ negative self-talk after missing days of activity. Although autonomous motivation is preferred, both types of motivation have a place within an MI session.

Autonomous Motivation

Autonomous motivation is present when one is motivated by either the inherent satisfaction of an activity or task or its alignment with his core values. If an individual is driven primarily by autonomous motivation then his motivation comes from within, absent from any outside pressure. Higher amounts of this motivation are associated with an increase in sustained behavior change (Landry & Solmon, 2004).

An exerciser fueled by autonomous motivation may:

- Hit the gym because she knows that doing so will improve her overall mood and decrease the stress from a hard workday.
- Try to set a new personal record for pull-ups or lap times in the pool.
- Arrange a game of beach volleyball to enjoy time with friends in the warm sun.
- Make a goal to do something active each day of the week because he feels sluggish, tired, and slightly depressed if he doesn't.
- Sign up to run a race for charity because it gives her a personal goal and aligns with her values of health and serving others.

Exercise produces many potentially life-enhancing intrinsic benefits and can easily be interesting and engaging. Joining a softball team after work, hiking on the weekends with friends, skiing, biking, dancing, and gardening are all examples of activities that exercise your body but are also fun and engaging.

There are more than 60 documented benefits to physical activity, many of which are considered intrinsic. Physical activity has the potential to elevate your mood, reduce stress, and give you a sense of accomplishment. It can be fun and pleasurable no matter what effect it has on your physical appearance. Clients are often aware of the physical health benefits of exercise but are unaware of the intrinsic, mood-enhancing benefits. By tuning clients in to the immediate positive effects exercise can have on mental and emotional health, they may become more motivated to fit it into their busy lives. For example, when a client notices that riding her bike to work instead of driving actually puts her in a better mood when she gets home, she may be more likely to select this form of transportation. You can ask permission to communicate the intrinsic benefits of exercise with your clients in order to help them build habits that will stand the test of time.

To help clients shift focus to autonomous motivation, ask them how being active aligns with their beliefs and values. Invite them to explore how they feel before, during, and after exercising. Reflect and summarize change talk that emphasizes the life-enhancing qualities of physical activity. It may also be appropriate to find out how previous attempts at being active failed to meet the client's expectations.

> *Reflect and summarize change talk that emphasizes the life-enhancing qualities of physical activity.*

Handout 14.1 outlines how clients can start to tune into intrinsic rewards of physical activity. In the spirit of MI, ask the client how being active influences mood, sleep patterns, and overall well-being. If your client is unaware of the many intrinsic benefits that are tied to physical activity, ask for permission to share a list. Invite the client to express which intrinsic benefits are important to him.

The term *intuitive exercise* has been used to describe focusing on how the body feels when physically active and is powered by optimism, self-trust, and the pleasure experienced in seeking adventure with physical activity (Tribole & Resch, 2012). A good way to help your clients make the shift to intuitive exercise is to invite them to brainstorm enjoyable activities or strategies for changing their current plan to make it more enjoyable. Emphasizing "fun" naturally changes the motivation to exercise. No longer is the focus predominately on managing blood sugar or fitting into a new pair of jeans; the focus is on spending your time doing something fun that is also physically active.

A client could be encouraged to go for a run or walk in the park on a spring day when the trees are blooming or grab a friend during a lunch break and power walk while they catch up on each other's lives. They could also sign up for a fun run/walk fundraiser with a group of friends, join a running club, garden, or simply take their kids outside and join in on a game of hide-and-seek, instead of just watching them play. These are just a few of the many ideas that a community may offer. Get to know the low-cost and fun activities in your area and make up a circle chart of ideas for your clients to choose from. Tapping into your client's inner, happy self will make exercise a sustainable and non-negotiable part of life. (See Chapter 3 for more information about circle charts.)

> *In the spirit of MI, ask the client in what ways being active influences mood, sleep patterns, and overall well-being.*

Here are some open-ended questions and reflections that could help your clients consider the intrinsic benefits of physical activity:

FITNESS THAT LASTS A LIFETIME:
INTRINSIC MOTIVATIONS FOR PHYSICAL ACTIVITY

You've probably heard that exercise is good for you, but you may not be aware of the many ways being active can not only improve your health, but improve your life. In fact, there at least 60 documented benefits of physical activity. Some benefits are noticed right away, either during the activity or immediately after.

Researchers have discovered that people who are more aware of the intrinsic motivations (motivations that come from within) are more likely to consistently include physical activity into their week. No medication or pill can provide the long list of intrinsic benefits that you may experience when you simply move your body. Here's a list of the immediate benefits many exercisers notice.

Being physically active . . .

- Increases energy levels.
- Produces a sense of accomplishment or empowerment.
- Improves sleep patterns.
- Intensifies hunger signals throughout the day.
- Reduces feelings of stress and anxiety.
- Results in fewer body aches and pains (low to moderate intensity).
- Improves sensitivity to the body's own insulin, immediately improving blood sugar control.
- Improves self-esteem.
- Improves body image.
- Increases mental focus.
- Increases strength and stamina.
- Decreases depression and stress levels.
- Improves digestion.
- Increases flexibility.
- Alleviates menstrual cramps.
- Enhances coordination and balance.
- Increases range mobility and range of motion.

Overall, being physically active feels good, improving mood and disposition. Which of these benefits have you already noticed?

_____

_____

Which of these benefits would you like to pay closer attention to next time you are physically active?

_____

_____

Based on Mahle Lutter, Rex, Hawkes, and Bucaccio (1999).

"What do you enjoy about your time walking in the park?"

"How does your body feel when you are active? During? After?"

"Exercise makes you feel energized."

"You are better prepared to deal with the stress at work on the days you go to the gym in the morning."

"You are more in touch with your hunger cues on the days you are active."

"You can tell that when you're active you feel fewer body aches and pains."

"How do your blood sugars run on the days when you're active?"

"How does being active influence your mood?"

"You've noticed being active helps you manage depression."

In an effort to become more intuitive exercisers, some clients benefit from keeping an exercise feelings journal (Handout 14.2) for a short period of time. In order to properly complete the log, clients focus on how they feel in the moment. So often, people exercise and disassociate themselves from the present moment. It can be in order to deal with the boredom of monotonous movements, numb themselves from aches and pains, or to ignore fatigue among other things. "Zoning out" or "checking out" in an attempt to distract from the uncomfortable sensations of a specific activity makes it difficult to tune into the positive rewards as well. If a particular activity is only tolerable if distracted from his or her own body, then it's probably not the kind of activity that fully engages and provides enough intrinsic reward to be sustainable.

No longer is the focus predominately on managing blood sugar or fitting into a new pair of jeans; the focus is on spending your time doing something enjoyable that is also physically active.

In the following example, a health coach discusses exercise with a client using motivational interviewing in a way that supports intrinsic motivation and autonomy.

PRACTITIONER: How do you feel about being physically active? [open-ended question]

CLIENT: I know I need to exercise more. [change talk] I was going for walks in the afternoon [change talk] but it has been so cold lately, so I've stopped. [sustain talk]

PRACTITIONER: You'd like to figure out ways to be active that aren't influenced by the weather. [simple reflection that emphasizes change talk] What other reasons, if any, caused you to stop? [open-ended question]

EXERCISE FEELINGS JOURNAL

Use this journal to record your physical activity patterns for a few days. By writing down your activity patterns and associated feelings, you may become more aware of the immediate benefits experienced following a session of exercise. Focus on the physical and emotional sensations you experience before, during and after the activity. Try to identify activities that are engaging, leave you feeling good, and are fun.

Date/Time: _May 8th, 12:30 pm_
Exercise Description: _Brisk walking for 25 min. during lunch break with_
    a coworker
Feelings Before: _Mentally exhausted and frustrated_
Feelings During: _Out of breath at times but not intolerable. Warm sun and fresh_
    air felt good
Feelings After: _Less frustrated and eager to make some progress on the mountain_
    of work in front of me

Date/Time: _____

_____

Exercise Description: _____

_____

Feelings Before: _____

_____

Feelings During: _____

_____

Feelings After: _____

_____

Date/Time: _____

_____

Exercise Description: _____

_____

Feelings Before: _____

_____

Feelings During: _____

_____

Feelings After: _____

_____

CLIENT: Honestly, it felt like a chore. I would just rather not. [sustain talk]

PRACTITIONER: It was something you made yourself do but you weren't getting any enjoyment out of it. And now that the weather is better, you're finding it hard to get going again. [reflection of sustain talk]

CLIENT: Yes, but I don't know what else to do. I can't afford to join a gym. [sustain talk]

PRACTITIONER: Money is another factor. [reflection of sustain talk] Tell me about a time when you enjoyed being physically active, if that's ever been the case? [evoking change talk]

CLIENT: I used to be very active when I was younger. I'd walk for an hour in the morning just to get outside and breathe in the fresh air.

PRACTITIONER: It sounds like you used to really enjoy your walks. What changed for you? Why does it feel like a chore now? [open-ended question]

CLIENT: I'm not comfortable like I used to be. I was thin then.

PRACTITIONER: Exercising felt good because you weren't self-conscious about your body. [complex reflection] What about going for a walk makes you feel self-conscious now? [open-ended question]

CLIENT: I just feel like everyone's looking at me and thinking about how much weight I've gained. I know I shouldn't care about what they think, but it just bothers me.

PRACTITIONER: You've stopped doing something that you used to really enjoy because you're afraid of what people may or may not be thinking about you. [complex reflection] What do you think about that? [open-ended question]

CLIENT: It sounds stupid. I really don't even run into people I know when I go on a walk. [change talk]

PRACTITIONER: It doesn't sound logical to you. [simple reflection] I wonder if you had something else to think about or focus on while walking you wouldn't worry about what other people are thinking. When you used to walk, what did you like to think about? [open-ended question]

CLIENT: I just liked feeling strong. I would go out in the morning when the air is crisp and push myself to do more than I did before. [change talk]

PRACTITIONER: You felt powerful during your walks, like you had accomplished something when you were done. I bet doing it in the morning set you up for a good day too. [reflection of change talk]

CLIENT: Yeah, it usually would. I'm far more organized when I get up in the morning. Plus I sleep better when I have a routine and make myself get up. [change talk]

PRACTITIONER: Working out was never really about how you looked, but more about how it made you feel. You felt powerful and accomplished; you got a jump on the day and felt more organized; plus, you slept better, giving you more energy the next day. Physical activity did a lot of positive things for you, but now the thought that people might think less of you is getting in the way of you feeling good about yourself. [summarizing change talk] What do you think? [open-ended question]

CLIENT: I guess so. I just don't know how to get over that hurdle. It gets in my way every time. I have really good intentions and then each time I try to do it, it gets harder and harder. [sustain talk]

PRACTITIONER: You're looking for ways to overcome those hurdles. [continuing the paragraph reflection, taking a guess at change talk] I have some ideas if you'd like to hear them. [asking permission]

CLIENT: Yes.

PRACTITIONER: People tend to feel inspired to exercise when they focus on the way being active makes them feel. You might find you enjoy it more when you are more focused on how you feel instead of losing weight. Some things to notice might be your breathing, how your muscles move, and how your energy level increases. Just like before, you would smell the crisp air and enjoy your surroundings in the morning. [provide (giving information)] What do you think of this information? [elicit]

CLIENT: I like that. I think I have been too wrapped up in my head that I'm not enjoying the process. It might even be fun to call up one of my girlfriends and ask her to go with me. [change talk]

PRACTITIONER: Going with a friend can help you get started again. [reflection of change talk]

CLIENT: I think we'd have a really good time.

PRACTITIONER: Having a friend with you will help you enjoy the time more. [simple reflection] Some of my clients have found that jotting down the feelings they notice before, during, and after an activity helps them to be more mindful of the process. I have an activity journal here [Handout 14.2] if that's something that you think might be helpful. What do you think? [elicit]

CLIENT: Yes, I can take that. I may not fill it out, but it will remind me to pay attention to those things.

PRACTITIONER: You like the idea of shifting your focus to enjoying the walk with a friend and noticing how being active in that way makes you feel. The cold weather is a barrier for you in the winter that really robs you of the joy of moving your body. If you're interested, we can talk more about indoor activities next time. For now, you've expressed an interest in some regular walks with your friend paired with mindfulness of your emotions and energy before, during, and after each walk. [summary]

Controlled Motivation

Exercise goals made from controlled motivation reflect an outward gain or payoff. This payoff or reward could be external, like attempting to lose 5 pounds because you believe doing so will impress former classmates at a high school reunion. However, it could also be internal, such as going to an exercise class to avoid the anxiety or guilt about choosing not to attend. What makes these two examples similar is the sense that the person is not making the decision free from pressure or negativity. An individual motivated primarily by controlled motivation exercises to avoid feelings of guilt, compete with others, or to reach a certain calorie burn or dress size (Deci & Ryan, 2008).

An exerciser acting from controlled motivation might:

- Compete in a sport in order to win and impress other people.
- Choose a certain series of abdominal exercises for the sole purpose of muscle definition.
- Buy herself a coffee drink as a reward for going to the gym all week.
- Only exercise to lose weight for a wedding and then stop exercising when the wedding is over.
- Only allow himself to have a 300-calorie meal if he burns 300 calories according to his heart rate monitor device.
- Go to an exercise class because she will feel guilty and anxious if she skips it.

Setting up external rewards for physical activity is not inherently bad. In fact, it is often the initial dominant form of motivation when clients begin an exercise routine. It may be helpful, at first, for the client to set up a reward system to get started. Using MI, the conversation may sound something like this:

PRACTITIONER: Some of my clients have found it helpful to set up a reward system when getting started with a new activity plan. Would you be interested in hearing more about this strategy? [asking permission]

CLIENT: Yes, that might help.

PRACTITIONER: There are many ways to do it, and you can decide what might work best for you. [supporting autonomy] One way is to set a weekly goal such as going for a walk three days a week. And then for each week you are successful in reaching that goal, you treat yourself to an inexpensive reward, such as a magazine in the grocery store checkout line or downloading a new song to listen to. Others prefer setting up rewards based on total minutes or steps per week or per month. [giving information] What do you think of this approach? [elicit]

CLIENT: I like that. I love going to the movies, so I think I'll take myself to the movies at the end of the month if I've met my monthly goal. Maybe I could set a monthly goal of going for a walk 12 times.

PRACTITIONER: You found something that could get you excited about your new plan.

However, if controlled motivation remains the dominant force, it is more than likely to waver, especially once the external reward is removed (Deci, Koestner, & Ryan 1999). This is seen in employee wellness programs that offer financial incentives for increasing physical activity. It can be the catalyst that gets people active, but it also can result in employees focusing only on the reward and not the intrinsic benefits of the physical activity.

When clients focus only on external rewards and feel that they are not totally free to make their own decisions, the activity becomes unsustainable. To illustrate this further, consider the following example:

Tracie, a part-time bank teller and mother of two children is starting an aerobics class with her friend Jessica. She feels compelled to join the class because Jessica wants to lose weight and has asked Tracie to help by going with her to the class. If it were entirely up to her, Tracie would do something outside of the gym that included her family.

Tracie is motivated by the desire to support her friend, and she would feel guilty if she didn't try to help. They do a few weeks of the class together and Tracie isn't very good at it. She feels unskilled and uncoordinated, leaving her feeling slightly humiliated. After 2 weeks Jessica gets a cold and cancels. Tracie then doesn't go by herself and never gets back into it.

Both Tracie's and Jessica's motivation would be categorized as controlled. Jessica was exercising for the external reward of perceived weight loss, and Tracie was stuck in an activity she didn't really enjoy and was only going to support her friend.

Figure 14.1 highlights some of the common extrinsic reinforcers that motivate people to be physically active. Although these may be the reasons

- Monetary rewards for reaching personal activity goals.
- Rewards from winning a competition (honors, trophies, etc.).
- Changes to physique (weight loss, muscle tone, weight gain, etc.).
- Pressure from friends or family.
- Compliments from friends or family.
- Money or incentive for physical activity.
- Rewards for attendance to a workout class or sport practice.
- Punishment for missing a workout class or sport practice.
- Improved lab values such as cholesterol, blood sugars, and blood pressure.
- Decreased risk of disease.

FIGURE 14.1. Common extrinsic motivators for physical activity.

why people start exercising, it is important to help clients make a shift from initially focusing on an external reward to realizing the intrinsic benefits.

In fact, when people are given external rewards for activities that are intrinsically interesting, the amount of intrinsic motivation regrettably diminishes (Deci et al., 1999). Other factors that decrease intrinsic motivation are the threat of punishment (Deci & Cascio, 1972), surveillance (Plant & Ryan, 1985), evaluation (Deci & Ryan, 2008), and negative feedback (Vellerand & Reid, 1984).

SELF-EFFICACY AND EXERCISE

Adopting a new physical activity routine can be daunting, especially if the client is hoping to explore a new sport or style of exercise. For some, the risks of looking silly, having poor coordination, or being uncomfortable can be enough to scare them away from trying fun and physically challenging activities.

Even if a person doesn't yet have the skill to master a particular activity, with time and perseverance, the skills often develop and more of the intrinsic benefits surface. The question, though, is how to help clients to persevere through the awkward initial trial period when starting a new activity.

The answer is found in building client *self-efficacy*, otherwise known as self-confidence in one's abilities for a specific task or activity. For example, a client may have high self-efficacy for running after being on the high school cross-country team, but have low self-efficacy for tennis. Therefore, when clients start new activities, they will commonly have low self-efficacy. To help them get over this hump, emphasize "starting small." Urge your clients to set up goals they feel confident in meeting. A good scaling question can help you gauge their readiness and confidence: "On a scale of 0 to 10, with 0 being not confident at all and 10 being 100% confident, how confident are you that you can correctly use the strength-training machines at the gym?" If the client reports low confidence, discuss ways to increase self-efficacy, such as meeting with a personal trainer, going with a friend who knows how to use the machines, or finding instructional videos online.

Guide your client to come up with a small, manageable goal. No goal is too small for the purpose of increasing self-efficacy. Perhaps your client sets a simple goal of asking a friend to join him at the gym. The main goal is to help your client find success, even if he reaches a very small goal. You can help your clients see their own potential when they accomplish small goals, and ultimately it will build their self-efficacy for maintaining the activity.

Other ways to build self-efficacy involve having your client examine his or her beliefs about what physical activity is and what it is not. Many clients have preconceived notions about physical activity that set them up to select unreasonable goals. For example, it is a common belief that physical activity only benefits you if it's continuous at a gym or an organized workout class. This is simply untrue. Small bouts of physical activity have been known to generate significant benefits as well. Once your clients realize that small amounts of physical activity spread throughout a typical week can improve health and well-being, they will be more willing to set smaller, more realistic goals. Handout 14.3 has examples of quick, easy ways clients can sneak physical activity into their week.

Before providing your clients with ideas for increasing physical activity, find out more about your clients' previous experiences. Be sensitive to their past experiences with exercise and dieting. There will be times when your clients may voice feeling intimidated or humiliated during certain activities. Those experiences and underlying beliefs about physical activity may be what have been keeping your client from being active up until now.

ADDRESSING BARRIERS TO BEING PHYSICALLY ACTIVE

Clients often cite many different barriers to being physically active on a regular basis. When researchers evaluated 56 structured exercise programs, they discovered that 50% of people who start exercising drop out within the first 6 months (Dishman, 1991). According to the Centers for Disease Control and Prevention (2014), 52% of adults do not meet the 2008 Physical Activity Guidelines. Figure 14.2 includes several commonly reported barriers to physical activity.

Like any behavior change, clients express ambivalence in their decision to start or continue exercising. Straightforward discussions about specific barriers can help clients evaluate what is keeping them from being active. The following are a few open-ended questions that could help you get started in discussing this topic:

Handout 14.3

FITTING IN FITNESS: CREATIVE WAYS
TO SQUEEZE PHYSICAL ACTIVITY INTO YOUR DAY

It's often challenging to find time to exercise. Many believe that exercise has to look a certain way or be a certain length in order for it to "count." The truth is that any time you move your body it counts as physical activity.

If you're feeling too busy to work out, consider incorporating these quick little bursts of physical activity into your day:

- Park in the farthest spot in the parking lot and walk.
- Take the stairs instead of the elevator/escalator.
- Take a 10-minute walk on your lunch break or during a rest period.
- Walk or bike to work, or drive halfway to work and walk or bike the rest of the way.
- Walk or bike to the store for light groceries.
- Take a stretch break every 2 hours to get your blood circulating.
- Walk around the perimeter of the field while your child is at a sports practice.
- Walk over to a coworker's office instead of calling, texting, or emailing to ask a question.
- Initiate walking meetings at work when meeting with two or three people.
- Walk to the mailbox instead of picking it up in the car on your way in or out of the driveway.
- Walk around the block with your family after dinner.
- When watching a television program do strength-building activities during the commercial break (such as push-ups or sit-ups).
- Clean the house or garden.
- Turn on some music and dance in your living room.

Which of the strategies above, if any, sound like feasible ways to add more activity to your day?

_____
_____
_____
_____

What other ideas do you have?

_____
_____
_____
_____

_____
Based on Kowalski (2010).

- Perceived lack of time.
- Perceived lack of convenience.
- Fear of injury.
- Poor self-efficacy.
- Unrealistic expectations.
- Negative self-talk.

FIGURE 14.2. Common barriers to consistent physical activity.

"What most concerns you about being physically active?"

"What tends to get in the way of being active?"

"How do you feel about being physically active?"

"If you decided to start working out tomorrow, what would need to happen?"

"When you see yourself being active, what kind of activities do you see yourself doing?"

"What's not working well with your current physical activity routine?"

Depending on the client's perceived barriers to being more physically active, a number of MI strategies can be used to evoke change talk and support the client in coming up with viable solutions. The following sections include an in-depth look at common barriers clients report to being physically active.

Perceived Lack of Time

The number-one barrier to being physically active in healthy adults is a perceived lack of time (Chinn, White, Harland, Drinkwater, & Raybould, 1999). People make time for the things that are important to them. It may be that your client has not made time for exercise before now, but would be able to if priorities changed. However, the perception of having no time has immobilized him. It can be helpful to explore this perception with your client to gain insight into how having no free time interacts with other possible barriers.

For example, having no free time may be linked to a belief that physical activity only counts if it is for 1 hour at the gym, 5 days a week. It is reasonable, therefore, for physical

People make time for the things that are important to them.

activity to be too time consuming for some. Alternatively, by exploring the preconceived notions of physical activity, you can clarify any misinformation and help your clients set goals that fit into their busy lives. The following script highlights a client and practitioner exploring physical activity while reviewing an exercise frequency questionnaire.

PRACTITIONER: It says here that you are physically active once a week, and you've written in the margin "if I'm lucky." What do you mean by "if I'm lucky"? [open-ended question]

CLIENT: Well, I have a lot going on. If everything comes together I'll be able to steal away to the gym for a while. But it rarely happens. I used to go three to five times a week before my husband and I had our kids.

PRACTITIONER: You have a pretty hectic schedule, which tends to push getting to the gym to the end of the list. [reflection]

CLIENT: It's not that it's not a priority for me. It's just that when I'm home in the evenings and the kids get home it's all homework and dinner. There's always something else that needs my attention.

PRACTITIONER: Physical activity would need to be something that fits easier into your life and involve your family. [reflection] If you were to start doing more activities that didn't impose on your family life, what would they be? [open-ended question]

CLIENT: Well, sometimes I take our dog for a walk. [change talk] It's usually my son's responsibility, but I do it when he's too busy with homework. Sometimes we do it together, but I don't break a sweat.

PRACTITIONER: Since you don't break a sweat, you're wondering if it still counts. [reflection]

CLIENT: It's just not the same as when I work out. We're just walking around and having fun.

PRACTITIONER: And when you think of exercise, you don't think about having fun. [reflection]

CLIENT: When I think of exercise, I think of sweating, like running or something.

It is no wonder the client has not made time to go to the gym. She doesn't connect exercise with enjoyment or pleasure. She sees exercise as a chore or a punishment. People rarely make time for things they hate, but if the activity could involve things she already loves doing and perhaps include the people she enjoys spending time with, she might find a physical activity she looks forward to doing. Furthermore, if practitioners can guide clients into breaking activities up into short bouts that easily fit within a busy schedule, clients may be more successful squeezing activity in during their regular routine.

Lack of Enjoyment

Many find exercise boring or tedious—something you have to do, but don't want to. Therefore, they sign up for a gym membership that goes unused as they voice many legitimate reasons why they can't go. The fact is, they have other more pressing issues, or they simply don't want to go, and that's OK.

Helping clients make fitness goals starts with finding out what they like to do. As with people, physical activity comes in many shapes and sizes; one size doesn't fit all. It is with this attitude that the spirit of MI comes alive in your counseling through the use of empathy. Expressing empathy means looking at a situation through your client's eyes and understanding how he or she would feel, not how you would feel in the same situation. Allow your clients the autonomy to come up with their own goals and ideas that make being active enjoyable.

Exacerbation of a Health Condition

Another common barrier that may arise revolves around the perception that exercise can have a negative effect on a certain disease or condition. For example, clients with type I diabetes may have trouble with low blood sugar (hypoglycemia) during vigorous workouts. The fear of hypoglycemia may be enough to discourage them from participating in routine physical activity. People who have had a heart attack, stroke, or are rehabilitating from orthopedic surgery are among those who may struggle with the fear of exacerbating their condition.

Clients tend to get stuck in three common traps when thinking about physical activity: (1) the all-or-nothing trap, (2) the guilt trap, and (3) the exercise as a punishment trap.

The All-or-Nothing Trap

Every year, January 1 comes around and New Year's resolutions start forming. People tend to expect themselves to be able to do more than they actually can or are willing to do. They make vague goals that focus more on extrinsic reward than the intrinsic process and give up when they don't see it going their way. For example, one such goal is with weight loss.

> Ted has been wanting to lose weight. He's being pushed by his wife and doctor to reduce his heart disease risk. He has high cholesterol, and it was recommended that he do some light physical activity on most days. Ted has been mostly sedentary for the past 2 years and elects to start jogging after work for 60 minutes and weighing himself weekly to track his progress. He decides to jog 5 days a week at the park near work. After 2 weeks he's exhausted and sore but excited to check in with the scale. Not only does Ted find that he has not lost weight, he has gained 2 pounds. He becomes discouraged and throws up his hands, saying, "I quit!" He feels bad about himself and fed up with trying to get healthier. His wife comes home, surprised to see Ted home so early, sitting on the couch watching a football game.

Ted fell into the all-or-nothing trap. He set himself up to do too much and had unrealistic expectations. On top of it, he saw himself getting further from his goal, so he quit. Alternatively, this could all have been avoided if someone had helped guide him toward a more specific, process-driven, intrinsically motivated goal from the start. At this point, Ted has no intrinsic motivation for being active. His extrinsic motivators are to lose weight and lower his cholesterol, which he believes will decrease his risk of developing heart disease. He is also extrinsically motivated as a result of the pressure he gets from both his wife and doctor. It's not unusual, therefore, for him to quit, especially when the extrinsic reward is removed. (He didn't see any weight loss.)

Let's start over at the beginning. Ted comes to you with orders from his doctor to lower his cholesterol and start doing some light physical activity on most days. Using MI, you can help guide Ted to make a goal that supports his doctor's orders and sets him up for a sustainable and intrinsically motivated healthy habit.

> PRACTITIONER: Hi, Ted, what brings you in to see me today? [open-ended engaging question]
>
> TED: My doctor told me to come see you. The last couple times I've seen him, he's been on me about my cholesterol. He thinks some exercise will help.
>
> PRACTITIONER: Your doctor is concerned about your cholesterol and had recommended you do some physical activity to help get it down. [simple reflection] What do you think about that plan? [open-ended question]
>
> TED: I think it's a great idea. I used to be pretty fit, but lately I've just gotten out of the habit.
>
> PRACTITIONER: You're pretty excited to get started and feel the way you used to when you were in shape. [reflection, taking a guess at unspoken change talk]
>
> TED: Yeah. I'm thinking about bringing my workout clothes to work and heading over the park for a jog before I go home. [change talk]
>
> PRACTITIONER: You've really thought about this and you're ready to start feeling better again. When you used to be fit you felt different. [reflection emphasizing change talk] How did you feel back then? [open-ended question that evokes change talk]
>
> TED: I had more energy. I felt good about myself. Strong. [change talk]
>
> PRACTITIONER: You were energized and confident. You want that back. [reflection emphasizing change talk]
>
> TED: Yes, I want to look in the mirror and see my old self again. [change talk]

PRACTITIONER: You want to see a person who's goal oriented and happy with a regular workout routine. [reflection of change talk] Take me through your plan. [open-ended question]

TED: OK. So I bring my workout clothes with me to work, change at the office, then drive over to the park. I'm thinking that an hour jog takes me around the entire loop three times. That's what I was doing before. [change talk]

PRACTITIONER: Three loops around the park or about an hour jog is your ultimate goal. [reflection of change talk] How confident are you on a scale of 0 to 10 that you'll be able to do three laps on your first day, with 0 being not confident and 10 being 100% confident? [scaling question]

TED: I think it's about a 7.

PRACTITIONER: How come a 7 and not an 8 or 9? [probing questions to explore possible barriers]

TED: It's been a while since I've been out jogging. I'm a little worried that I might not make it for the whole hour. [sustain talk] But any time is good, right?

PRACTITIONER: When you really think it through, you're seeing that 60 minutes sounds like a lot right off that bat, but you're willing to get out there and see what you can do. [complex reflection] What would you think about doing an experiment this week to ease in more gradually? [open-ended question]

TED: What do you have in mind?

PRACTITIONER: One idea is to take this week and go through the motions to make sure you've got everything set up right. Maybe just put on your clothes at work and head to the park. You could jog a little if you feel like it, but set the goal of just "showing up" this week. Then maybe next week, after you've played around with this part of the goal, you could set a certain number of minutes or laps that line up with your current fitness level. Some of my clients have found it useful to use this fitness journal when getting started to write down your activity and how it feels each time you go. [giving information] What do you think? [elicit]

TED: I like this. I can do this each day this week and let you know how it goes when I come in next week. [change talk]

PRACTITIONER: You're feeling more confident. How confident are you on that scale from 0 to 10, now that we've readjusted your goal? [scaling question]

TED: Now I'm a 9 or maybe even a 10!

Ted came in with some pretty high expectations for himself. The practitioner used a scaling question to see how confident Ted was in his goal and found he had some reservations. The counselor was able to suggest a fitness journal to help Ted gauge his abilities and gave him the permission to alter his goal as he went. This technique ultimately supports Ted in making goals that go at his own pace. Next week he'll be likely to have experienced some success, since his goal was developed around the process instead of the outcome.

The Guilt Trap

The all-or-nothing trap tends to transform into the guilt trap. When clients perceive they have not met their goal for the day, instead of brushing themselves off and starting anew, they throw in the towel and say, "I just can't do this," "I'm not worth it," "Why did I think I could do this in the first place?" This negative self-talk breeds a mindset of failure and squashes any motivation that recently sprouted.

When a client comes back to you feeling dejected and discouraged, explore the guilt and shame she may be experiencing. She may think the guilt-filled thoughts will ultimately motivate her to restart. By asking a good evoking question, you may be able to help her recognize the damaging nature of negative self-talk. For example, you could ask, "How might the guilt you are experiencing for not reaching your goal keep you from starting up again?" By using some CBT in combination with MI, you may be able to tune your client into the unhelpful nature of negative self-talk and guide her to come up with positive self-talk replacements.

CBT is the practice of changing your thoughts to create a chain reaction that ultimately changes how you feel, how you act, and the results you see (Beck, 2005). If your client is able to change her thought from "I just can't do this," to "I sometimes have a hard time with this," she might be more inclined to start up again. Instead of "I feel lousy and guilty," she could reframe the statement to, "I could try that again but with a little less of this and that and a little more of these." The key is to help your client become aware of the negative self-talk and guide her in developing positive self-talk replacements. She will be more likely to try again and then enjoy the results of accomplishing her goal.

You can help her make those changes by asking open-ended questions about her negative self-talk, reflecting her feelings, and asking permission before offering alternative positive self-talk.

The Exercise as a Punishment Trap

Many people use exercise as a way to make up for undesirable eating behaviors. The old adage of energy balance described as energy in = energy out becomes a construct that can oversimplify the very complex variables of metabolism and appetite. However, clients often get caught up in the thought that our bodies are simple math equations; if you burn a certain number of calories, you can erase that slice of cheesecake or milkshake. The truth is, counting calories you consume and charting the calories you burn rarely gives you reliable results after the first 6 months (Mann et al., 2007). Over time, people end up feeling discouraged and dreading the pre-scribed exercise as if it were a punishment for their eating "sins."

Clients can benefit more from nutrition and fitness counseling that is free from authoritative pressure. The right to eat what's right for your body is inalienable. No matter one's weight, there is nothing one can eat that is deserving of punishment. When the eating culture becomes one of sins and virtue, the cornerstone of well-being begins to crumble. No matter what kind of practitioner you are, you can help your clients see their inherent value as human beings and the potential they have to flourish. Because in the end, eating right and living an active lifestyle are only tools to improve and enhance one's ability to feel joy and live a happy life. Motivating one-self with guilt and shame rarely leads to happy and healthy living.

Through applying MI to a session about physical activity, the focus is shifted away from telling clients recommended minutes and steps neces-sary for good health and toward eliciting intrinsic motivation and enjoyable ways to move their bodies. In today's fast-paced world, it can be a challenge to find time to squeeze in physical activity. However, clients will go to great lengths to make time for activities that are fun and feel good. Self-discoveries of the life-enhancing properties of physical activity will result in a lifetime commitment to change.

CHAPTER 15

Putting Motivational Interviewing to Work to Address Weight Concerns and Disordered Eating

The scale can only give you a numerical reflection of your relationship with gravity. That's it. It cannot measure beauty, talent, purpose, life force, possibility, strength, or love.
—STEVE MARABOLI

We live in a dieting culture, bombarded daily by advertisements for weight loss aids with enticing success stories plastered on magazines, websites, and social media. From boot camp-style workout regimens, to commercial diet programs, diet pills, shakes, and surgeries, the message runs deep—beauty and health are dependent on body shape and size. And yet, more often than not, these attempts at losing weight fail (Mann et al., 2007).

The weight loss and diet control market is a $61 billion industry that is failing the American public (Market Data Enterprises, 2013). Weight loss programs, whether fad diets or under the guise of "lifestyle changes," are often chosen as short-term solutions, resulting in weight loss followed by weight regain (Bacon et al., 2002; Bacon, Stern, Van Loan, & Keim, 2005; Dansinger, Gleason, Griffith, Selker, & Schaefer, 2005; Dansinger, Tatsioni, Wong, Chung, & Balk, 2007; Mann et al., 2007; Neumark-Sztainer et al., 2006; Stice, Cameron, Killen, Hayward, & Taylor, 1999).

The weight loss and diet control market is a $61 billion industry that is failing the American public.

Weight loss programs are not only ineffective in the long run but also can be physiologically and psychologically damaging (Bacon et al., 2002; Bacon et al., 2005; Mann et al., 2007; Steinhardt, Bezner, & Adams, 1999; Tomiyama, Ahlstrom,

& Mann, 2013). Moreover, an individual's fitness level may be a better predictor of mortality than weight and body composition (Barry, Beets, Durstine, Liu, & Blair, 2014)

Emerging research suggests that promoting weight loss may cause more harm than good (Ramos Salas, 2015; Tylka et al., 2014); however, health care professionals are increasingly pressured to instruct their clients to lose weight. While practitioners have good intentions, they may be inadvertently promoting weight bias, which negatively affects their larger clients (Tomiyama, 2014). In fact, clients who are told to lose weight are more likely to gain weight over time (Sutin & Terracciano, 2013).

Weight bias can be defined as the inclination to form unreasonable judgments based on a person's weight (Washington, 2011). According to the Centers for Disease Control and Prevention (Washington, 2011), weight bias is caused by the belief that stigma and shame motivates people to lose weight. Weight bias often goes unnoticed due to cultural values of thinness. Thin is viewed as healthy and fat is viewed as unhealthy. In reality, size is not a direct reflection of health. Given the genetic component of body size, there are many thin individuals who are aerobically unfit and eat a nutrient-poor diet and many fat individuals who are aerobically fit and eat a nutrient-rich diet. Recent research comparing mortality rates among all weight categories has uncovered that your overweight and obese clients (body mass index = 25–35) may actually live the longest (Flegal, Kit, Orpana, & Graubard, 2013; Lantz, Golberstein, House, & Morenoff, 2010).

> *Motivating through shame and stigma is in direct opposition to the spirit of MI.*

Regardless of your clients' weight or health status, motivating them through shame and stigma is in direct opposition to the spirit of MI. True acceptance is modeled through communicating absolute worth no matter the clients' size or shape. The purpose of this chapter is to give you tools to discuss your clients' weight and disordered eating concerns with the spirit of MI as your guiding force and with the focus of your counseling on overall health and well-being. Whether your clients are struggling with binge-eating disorder, bulimia, or general body dissatisfaction, they will benefit from counseling that aims to heal their relationship with food and fitness while enhancing body esteem.

INTRODUCING A WEIGHT-NEUTRAL APPROACH

If improving health is truly the focus within a nutrition and fitness counseling session, then it is in the client's best interest for the practitioner to focus on nutrition and fitness behaviors and not on weight. The ultimate goal is for clients to make sustainable changes and mounting evidence suggests that a non-diet approach is more conducive to adopting long-term changes while minimizing disordered eating patterns (Tylka et al., 2014). In addition, this nonjudgmental, nonstigmatizing approach is preferred by clients, resulting in more return visits (Schaefer & Magnuson, 2014; Thomas, Lewis, Hyde, Castle, & Komesaroff, 2010).

One such non-diet approach is the Health At Every Size® (HAES®) paradigm (Figure 15.1).* The HAES approach differs from traditional weight-focused paradigms in that clients are encouraged to tune in to hunger and fullness cues, energy levels, and cravings to guide eating and activity timing and quantity (Bacon & Aphramor, 2011; Association for Size Diversity and Health, 2014). HAES is a weight-neutral approach, meaning that the focus is not on weight, but on helping the client make healthy lifestyle changes while allowing weight to stabilize at a number that is largely genetically driven and varies widely from person to person. Historically, the word "fat" has had a negative connotation; supporters of this movement advocate reclaiming this word as a descriptive term and not as a negative judgment of character or physicality.

Poor health and disease affects individuals of all sizes. The HAES message is not that all body weights are health-enhancing for all individuals. Not everyone is at a weight that is optimal for their health. However, that

---

1. **Weight inclusivity:** Accept and respect the inherent diversity of body shapes and sizes and reject the idealizing or pathologizing of specific weights.
2. **Health enhancement:** Support health policies that improve and equalize access to information and services, and personal practices that improve human well-being, including attention to individual physical, economic, social, spiritual, emotional, and other needs.
3. **Respectful care:** Acknowledge our biases, and work to end weight discrimination, weight stigma, and weight bias. Provide information and services from an understanding that socioeconomic status, race, gender, sexual orientation, age, and other identities impact weight stigma, and support environments that address these inequities.
4. **Eating for well-being:** Promote flexible, individualized eating based on hunger, satiety, nutritional needs, and pleasure, rather than any externally regulated eating plan focused on weight control.
5. **Life-enhancing movement:** Support physical activities that allow people of all sizes, abilities, and interests to engage in enjoyable movement, to the degree that they choose.

FIGURE 15.1. The Health At Every Size (HAES) principles. From the Association for Size Diversity and Health (2014). Reprinted by permission.

---

*Health At Every Size and HAES are registered trademarks of the Association for Size Diversity and Health and used with permission.

	Diet Paradigm	Non-Diet Paradigm
Food	• Food is labeled as good or bad. • Quantity and quality of food is determined by *external* source such as calories, grams, or exchanges.	• *All* food is acceptable. • Quantity and quality of food is determined by responding to *physical* cues such as hunger, fullness, taste, cravings, and body comfort.
Physical Activity	• Exercise to lose weight.	• Aim to be more active in fun and enjoyable ways.
Weight	• Define a goal weight.	• The body will seek its natural weight when individuals eat in response to internal physical cues.

FIGURE 15.2. Diet paradigm versus non-diet paradigm.

doesn't mean that attempting to lose weight is the answer, given the physical and emotional turmoil that often results. Across the weight spectrum, clients can aim to adopt eating and activity patterns that enhance physical and emotional health, regardless of changes in weight.

A key component of counseling using a non-diet approach is conveying an attitude of acceptance of size and shape differences and respecting and celebrating size diversity. This is done through inviting the client to explore emotional and physiological consequences of previous dieting attempts while at the same time exposing the client to a non-diet approach.

HAES messages are very different from traditional weight loss programs. Some of these key differences are summarized in Figure 15.2. Clients' reception of HAES principles depends heavily on the counseling style in which they are offered. If the information is provided using the various motivational interviewing techniques discussed throughout this book, the client will be far more receptive to this alternative way of thinking about food and fitness.

APPLYING THE HAES PRINCIPLES IN AN MI SESSION

The HAES paradigm is defined by the following five principles: weight inclusivity, health enhancement, respectful care, eating for well-being, and life-enhancing movement (Association for Size Diversity and Health, 2014). The remaining sections address each principle and include tips for providing nutrition and fitness counseling in a weight-neutral, nonstigmatizing manner that aligns with the spirit of MI.

Principle 1: Weight Inclusivity

The first HAES principle is to "accept and respect the inherent diversity of body shapes and sizes and reject the idealizing or pathologizing of specific weights." Clients seeking nutrition and fitness counseling often present with significant body dissatisfaction. The media contributes greatly to this dissatisfaction, with unrealistic images of beauty and the message that women must be thin and men must be muscular to be attractive, successful, and healthy. It is no surprise, then, that exposure to media is positively correlated with body dissatisfaction (Richins, 1991).

However, messages about weight and size also come from peers, parents, coaches, teachers, and relatives. It's important to explore the root of the client's body dissatisfaction within the context of a counseling session by asking open-ended questions, reflecting, and summarizing what you hear.

Messages from others about weight and body shape are typically received through direct and indirect communication. Often, clients will share stories of shaming comments made by parents during their formative years. Statements like, "Gosh, you've really filled out!" or "If you just watch what you eat, you could lose the weight you've gained," are all too common. Family members also indirectly model unhealthy behaviors such as dieting. They might weigh themselves regularly and make negative comments about their own physical appearance, setting their children up to do the same. Whether indirect or direct, these communicated messages can play a significant role in an individual's feelings about his or her own body.

One way to begin addressing your client's weight concerns is to invite him to share where the desire for changing his body shape or size comes from. Ask the client to share messages received about weight and shape while growing up in order to shed light on the client's current personal beliefs and how it relates to feelings of self-worth.

Here are open-ended questions that can evoke thoughts and feelings about weight and body image:

"What do you hope will improve if you weigh less?"

"What is it about your body that you don't like?"

"How do you feel about your body on a scale from 0 to 10, with 10 meaning you love your body and 0 meaning you hate it?"

"Describe the messages you heard about weight and size during your youth."

"How do your current negative feelings about your body size and shape relate to messages you've heard?"

"What are some negative messages about your body that come up for you during a typical day? How do these thoughts influence your food and fitness choices?"

"What are your thoughts when you step on the scale? How do those thoughts affect you during the day?"

Some clients believe that losing weight is the only way to improve their body image. In reality, losing weight does not always improve body image. On the other hand, sessions that include body image counseling can reduce body dissatisfaction (Rosen, Reiter, & Orosan, 1995). Body image counseling begins with having the client gain awareness of her negative body image, identify the negative self-talk surrounding body features, and find alternative positive self-talk statements to replace the old ones.

Larger individuals often feel that they have to change their bodies in order to be healthy, attractive, and comfortable in their own skin. However, feeling bad about your weight may be worse for your health than the weight itself (Latner, Durso, & Mond, 2013). Therefore, promoting a positive body image may improve health outcomes regardless of changes in body size.

Promoting a positive body image starts with the practitioner's attitude toward weight and size. The idea of having an unconditional positive regard for your client (discussed in Chapter 2) is communicated by emitting an aura of acceptance for the client's physical attributes regardless of weight loss. This undercurrent of acceptance is easily felt within the client–counselor relationship and not only fosters trust but also models a positive self-talk.

> *Unconditional positive regard for your client is communicated by emitting an aura of acceptance for the client's physical attributes regardless of weight loss.*

Gaining proficiency and confidence in body image counseling requires extensive training and practice. Practitioners who do not feel equipped to provide body image counseling can still help their clients by noticing body dissatisfaction and making referrals to trained professionals. (See Appendix 1, "Making Referrals.")

In the following script, the practitioner uses MI to invite a male client to explore the birth of his body dissatisfaction and how it may negatively affect his current health patterns. While reading this dialogue, notice how a few well-placed evoking questions can help increase the client's awareness of his negative body image, and how it may be hurting rather than helping his overall health and well-being. Toward the end, the practitioner elicits change talk for jumping off the yo-yo diet bandwagon.

PRACTITIONER: You've already made some significant changes to the way you eat. You've said a couple things, though, that lead me to believe that you won't feel successful unless you lose a certain amount of weight. [probing for body dissatisfaction] What do you think? [open-ended question]

CLIENT: I need to lose 50 pounds.

PRACTITIONER: You have an exact number in mind. [simple reflection] Could you expand on that a bit? What is it about losing 50 pounds that feels important? [open-ended question]

CLIENT: I'm sick of being *obese*. I've been big all my life. I've had a few ups and downs, but I've been overweight for as long as I can remember. I take after my dad, I think. My mom was always signing me up for sports to try to keep my weight down and it sort of worked, but now I'm in my 30s and it's time to get real. The doctor said I'm going to end up dying of a heart attack if I don't do something about my weight. [change talk—need to change]

PRACTITIONER: You and your doctor had an intense conversation about your heart health. [simple reflection]

CLIENT: She told me my cholesterol was high and she thinks I might be prediabetic, but if I do something about it now I can stop it.

PRACTITIONER: You're thinking that your weight is to blame for your high cholesterol and blood sugars. [continuing the paragraph reflection] This message that you need to lose weight has come from a few different places, starting with your mother in childhood. [complex reflection] What sort of messages did you hear growing up about body weight, shape, and size? [evoking with an open-ended question]

CLIENT: I think it all started with my grandmother. I remember one time I was over at her house because she wanted to make me some pajamas. I remember her measuring my waist and then telling my mom I was twice as big as my cousin Jimmy and she couldn't make them for me because she didn't have enough fabric. I think I was 9 or 10. That was when I realized I was bigger than everyone else.

PRACTITIONER: That's when you started to think there was something wrong with you because of your size. You've heard it from your grandmother, your mom, and now your doctor. [summary]

CLIENT: I hear it every day. I've stopped going out to eat because I feel like people judge what I order. The other day a little girl pointed at me and asked her mom if I had a baby in my belly.

PRACTITIONER: That must have felt really uncomfortable. [expressing empathy] You're hoping that losing 50 pounds will protect you from feeling like there's something wrong with you. [complex reflection] Could I share with you a little about the research regarding weight and health? [asking permission]

CLIENT: Sure.

PRACTITIONER: Well, one thing we know from scientific research is that body size is largely influenced by genetics. You mentioned you take after your father's body type. Research shows that people are really good at losing weight, but not good at keeping it off because our body is actually designed to fight back in order to survive periods of starvation from an evolutionary standpoint. That's why dieters are always losing and regaining weight. Plus, many of my clients have found that even when they do lose weight, they may feel better about their bodies temporarily, but then new issues of body image and self-worth arise. [giving information] What do you make of this information? [eliciting the client's response with an open-ended question]

CLIENT: I know what you mean. I lost 45 pounds a few years ago when I went on a low-carbohydrate diet. But I'm back where I started. It's pretty frustrating. [change talk for a non-diet approach]

PRACTITIONER: Yes, it can be a roller-coaster ride. [metaphor reflection that emphasizes change talk] And the good news is that making changes to the way you eat can improve your health no matter what goes on with your weight. Plus, there are other ways to improve the way you feel about your body so you won't feel so vulnerable to comments strangers make. [giving information] How would you feel about exploring some of these alternative ways to improve your health and body image? [asking permission]

In this excerpt, the practitioner used some evoking questions to encourage the client to explore the root of his negative body image. The practitioner also provided some information to the client (with permission) regarding genetics, dieting, and body image. The practitioner validated the client's concerns through the use of powerful reflections and increased his awareness of the complexities of weight and body image. A final reflection was provided that emphasized the client's change talk for considering an alternative approach. At this point, the practitioner can continue to guide the client through this exploration (if doing so is within the practitioner's scope of practice) or provide a referral to a therapist who specializes in body image counseling. (See Appendix 1, "Making Referrals.")

Principle 2: Health Enhancement

The second HAES principle is "to support health policies that improve and equalize access to information and services, and personal practices that improve human well-being, including attention to individual physical, economic, social, spiritual, emotional, and other needs." This concept points to the necessity of expressing compassion for clients. An MI practitioner is not seeking self-gain, but seeking the betterment of his clients.

The HAES paradigm is a holistic approach where all components of wellness are considered important to the individual's health and overall well-being. Health is about more than just diet and exercise. There's spiritual health, emotional health, social health, intellectual health, environmental health, and occupational health, to name a few.

> *Health is about more than just diet and exercise.*

Clients often assume that dieting will improve physical health. That is certainly up for debate (Tomiyama, Ahlstrom, & Mann, 2013). What is plain to see though is that dieting can come at a cost to the other facets of health and well-being. For example, in order to maintain motivation to eat less and exercise more on a daily basis a client pins a particularly unflattering "before" picture of herself to the refrigerator. This way, every time she goes to the fridge to eat she is reminded of her body weight from before she started dieting. Since most dieters regain lost weight (Mann et al., 2007), it is likely that she will return to the same weight as in her picture but with even lower self-esteem. This cycle generates negative self-talk and results in body dissatisfaction adding to the toll on emotional health. When she decides not to meet up with old friends because she is embarrassed about her weight, she experiences the cost to her social health too.

In promoting health and human well-being, it may be useful to invite your clients to consider the unadvertised costs of dieting. Clients often show up with great enthusiasm and interest for starting a new diet plan. In the spirit of MI, clients have complete autonomy to begin whatever diet plan they'd like; however, practitioners can offer concerns with evidence-based information, if the client is interested. Here are some evoking questions that can encourage exploration into the risks of dieting and help provide a platform for eliciting change talk toward a wellness-focused approach:

> "Describe your dieting history. What diets have you tried and what worked and didn't work for you in the past?"
> "What was it about the last diet you tried that made it hard to stick to?"
> "What is it about this new diet you're considering that appeals to you?"
> "What concerns, if any, do you have about starting a new diet?"
> "What was the emotional cost, if any, of previous diets you've tried?"
> "How did previous diets negatively affect your social life?"
> "How does dieting influence your emotional health?"

Often clients won't be interested in hearing an alternative non-diet approach until they've expressed dissatisfaction with a dieting experience.

By guiding the client to explore the costs of dieting, the client may become more open to the holistic messages of the HAES paradigm. In the following dialogue the practitioner elicits previous failed attempts at weight loss, highlighting the negative impact of dieting on emotional health with reflections and summaries. The practitioner uses an E-P-E technique to present the client with a non-diet approach.

> PRACTITIONER: You shared that you tried [commercial weight loss program] and it worked at first but then wasn't something that worked for you in the long term. [simple reflection] What did you like and not like about that program? [open-ended question]
>
> CLIENT: I liked that I ate really well and I lost weight.
>
> PRACTITIONER: You felt good about your food choices and for a while it got you the result you were looking for. [simple reflection]
>
> CLIENT: Yes. People started talking about how skinny I looked.
>
> PRACTITIONER: You liked that others noticed. [simple reflection] What about that eating plan, if anything, didn't work for you? [open-ended question]
>
> CLIENT: Well it did work for me, for a while. I actually really liked it. I did it for about 3 months and, I don't know, I just fell off the wagon one day when I gained weight for no reason. Then I didn't want to go in for the weigh-in because I had blown it.
>
> PRACTITIONER: You expected your weight to keep going down. When it stopped you found yourself less motivated to work the program. [simple reflection] This time, you want to do something that feels more sustainable, something that doesn't make you feel like throwing in the towel part way through. [reflecting implied change talk].
>
> CLIENT: Yes, I guess you're right. That makes a lot of sense and is actually a pattern, now that I think about it. As long as I'm losing weight I keep up with my diet, but as soon as I stop losing, I feel like throwing in the towel and giving up.
>
> PRACTITIONER: You're not alone in feeling that way. Many of my clients have shared that very same experience. What foods, if any, were you missing while on your last diet? [open-ended question]
>
> CLIENT: Well, I wasn't perfect on my diet. I did eat certain foods on the naughty list once in a while, but the food I found myself craving the most was cake. I could never really find a low-calorie alternative for cake, so I was always blowing it every time I celebrated someone's birthday.
>
> PRACTITIONER: You experienced a lot of guilt while on your last diet. [complex reflection]

CLIENT: I really did. But it was the only thing that has worked for me.

PRACTITIONER: Overall, you noticed that you like the way your body feels when you eat well. At the same time, you don't like having to miss out on celebrations, or the guilt associated with eating dessert. You found that while on the diet program you had a negative relationship with the scale, which took an emotional toll. You're here today because you're looking for a different approach. [summary emphasizing the drawbacks of dieting and change talk] Does that sound about right? [closed-ended question]

CLIENT: Yes, that sums it up.

PRACTITIONER: May I share with you some of my philosophies about weight, health, and dieting that I think might help you? [asking permission]

CLIENT: Sure!

PRACTITIONER: You're not alone with your experiences with dieting. Most dieters lose weight and then gain it back. It's not you who failed; it's the diet that failed you. Making changes in your eating and exercise patterns is hard work, especially if those changes involve restricting certain pleasurable foods or activities. Research actually supports that the dieting process is a recipe for disaster. There's also research that supports an alternative approach to dieting called non-dieting. [giving information] What have you heard about the term non-diet? [elicit]

CLIENT: Nothing. But I have heard that crash diets don't work.

PRACTITIONER: You've noticed extreme weight loss measures are ineffective. [simple reflection] Can I tell you more about a non-diet approach? [asking permission]

CLIENT: Please do.

PRACTITIONER: In a non-diet approach, the focus is on eating in response to hunger, fullness, and cravings instead of counting calories or points. You tune into how your body feels and choose foods that make it feel the best and eating times that honor your hunger. This approach also involves taking the focus off of the scale and pounds lost, and instead focusing your attention on how your body feels eating certain foods and doing certain activities. By shifting the focus away from the variations in your weight, you can more easily tune into your body's wants and needs. This is a different approach to healthy eating. What do you make of it? [elicit]

In this dialogue, the practitioner asked the client to share negative thoughts and feelings about dieting. The client voiced some aspects of the diet program that were negative, and the practitioner reflected those pieces as the change talk. In this case, change talk is the language the client uses that suggests that the old way of doing things (dieting) isn't working. At times the practitioner took some guesses at some unspoken change talk using complex reflections. Her educated guesses were based on what she'd heard from previous dieting clients who were feeling restricted and unhappy. As a result, the client started to voice change talk for an alternative approach. The practitioner then used the E-P-E strategy to give the client a brief overview of a weight-neutral approach. She asked permission before giving information about the non-diet approach, provided the information, and then followed up the explanation with an open-ended question to check in with the client's thoughts and feelings in the light of her own experiences and beliefs. If the client is open to exploring a non-diet approach, she may begin shifting her focus away from weight loss and toward eating and activity strategies that enhance overall health and well-being.

Principle 3: Respectful Care

Providing respectful care is to "acknowledge our biases, and work to end weight discrimination, weight stigma, and weight bias." In addition, when one provides respectful care, information and services are offered "from an understanding that socioeconomic status, race, gender, sexual orientation, age, and other identities impact weight stigma, and support environments that address these inequities."

Assumptions made about weight by health care professionals can result in the misdiagnosis of problems and the wrong plan of care for thin and fat clients. Health care professionals see a fat patient and assume he or she doesn't eat well and is sedentary. This is a false assumption, as many fat patients are very fit and eat well. Some researchers have found that individuals in the overweight and obese BMI categories don't necessarily eat more calories than those in the "normal" weight category (Fang, Wylie-Rosett, Cohen, Kaplan, & Alderman, 2003). Most concerning, clients told to lose weight often avoid their doctors, thereby missing the opportunity for routine preventive screenings (Amy et al., 2006).

Conversely, health care professionals often see a thin person and assume he or she eats well and is physically active. Given the genetic contributors of body weight, size, health, and disease, this is a false assumption. By making assumptions about one's eating and activity patterns based on body size, health care professionals may inadvertently fail to discuss eating and activity patterns with their thin patients. Therefore, weight bias affects individuals across the weight spectrum.

The spirit of MI is present in the context of providing respectful care. In order to deliver care that exudes acceptance, absolute worth, and

Examine the obvious and subtle ways your clients might feel stigmatized.

autonomy, examine the obvious and subtle ways your clients might feel stigmatized. Consider the environment of your office or workspace and try to see it through the eyes of your clientele. Is the seating adequate and comfortable for people of various shapes and sizes? Choose chairs or couches that allow larger clients to shift and reposition as they share their stories, experiences, thoughts and feelings with you.

In addition, choose wall hangings with weight-neutral imagery. Having only pictures of thin, happy people sends the message that clients will only be happy or healthy when they are thin. Include images of people of various sizes and shapes. Does your office monitor clients' weight, waist circumference, or fat fold thickness with each appointment? Consider the necessity of monitoring these data weighed against the potential negative psychological effects on clients.

Finally, examine your own biases and make efforts to challenge them. The anti-fat attitudes of health care professionals are well documented (Johnston, 2012). In your attempt to care for your clients with compassion, demonstrating absolute worth, examine your counseling environment. Aim to create a comfortable, accepting, and inviting atmosphere for clients across the weight spectrum.

Principle 4: Eating for Well-Being

The fourth HAES principle promotes "flexible, individualized eating based on hunger, satiety, nutritional needs, and pleasure, rather than any externally regulated eating plan focused on weight control."

A non-diet approach, such as HAES, involves eating in response to physiological cues such as hunger, fullness, and a sense of well-being. Using internal cues to regulate food intake is also known as intuitive or mindful eating. This is very different from a restriction-based diet approach in which calories are counted and food is weighed and measured. Intuitive eating is about attending to body cues, allowing oneself to become gently hungry before eating, and eating until comfortably satisfied. In terms of deciding what to eat, individuals following a non-diet approach pay attention to eating in a way that feels good, both in terms of body function and taste.

At times, certain foods are selected because they are ideal for maintaining energy throughout the day or assist with bowel regularity. At other times, foods are selected due to the enjoyment factor or the simple pleasure in satisfying taste buds. In drawing the client's attention to these internal responses the client is able to focus on the intrinsic benefits of food choices.

Mindfulness with eating involves slowing down and simply noticing or becoming aware of yourself and your surroundings as well as the pleasure you are experiencing from the food. On the contrary, mindlessness often involves eating more than was originally desired and missing the pleasure that food brings.

When clients suffer from chronic conditions that require specific diet modifications, the intrinsic benefits of picking and choosing foods that honor well-being become most pronounced. For example, a client with a new diagnosis of lactose intolerance will find that the body gives feedback when the offending foods are eaten. The motivation to eat lactose-free, therefore, comes from wanting to continue to feel well and avoid discomfort. With conditions such as diabetes, the body may give more subtle cues such as symptoms associated with hypo- or hyperglycemia. For some conditions, such as high cholesterol, there may not be any obvious body signals when eating foods that worsen the condition, but the client can tune into other body cues to guide eating choices, such as fatigue or mood.

Whether the body responds with a siren or a whisper, tuning in to the physical sensations before, during, and after eating can help clients navigate the waters of what, when, and how much to eat. If the client is interested in using a journaling exercise to gain awareness of body cues and feelings, the food and feelings journal presented in Chapter 5 could be provided. There is still a place for educating the client on certain offending foods when attempting to manage a disease or condition; however, by combining food knowledge with body awareness, the client may be more motivated to choose foods that make him feel better in the moment.

In a non-diet approach, clients aren't told how much or when to eat. Instead they are encouraged to become experts of their own body cues and nutritional needs. Clients are given full autonomy and are respected for their differences. In creating a partnership between the client and practitioner, the client is treated as the expert of his body and body cues. In the following dialogue, the practitioner shares a few insights about hunger and fullness, invites the client to focus on a topic of interest, and then guides the client toward beginning the journey of mindful eating.

CLIENT: Have you ever heard of a food coma? That's how I feel in the evenings. I do fine all day long, but once I eat dinner it's like opening the floodgates. I don't know how to stop it. I wish I could just push away my plate like my kids do. [change talk—desire to change]

PRACTITIONER: You don't like the way you feel so stuffed after dinner. And it also sounds like you're interested in exploring a new approach with me today. [reflection of change talk] If it's all right with you, I'd like to show you some different topics we could discuss today. [Handout 15.1]. [asking permission] Each circle includes strategies for eating more mindfully.

CIRCLE CHART FOR HUNGER AND FULLNESS

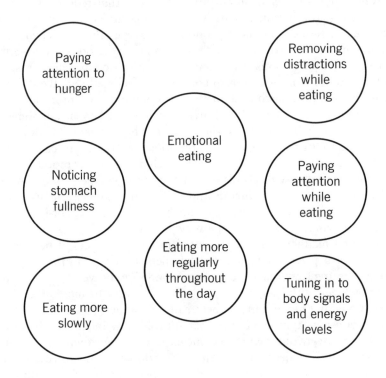

Paying attention to hunger

Removing distractions while eating

Emotional eating

Noticing stomach fullness

Paying attention while eating

Eating more regularly throughout the day

Eating more slowly

Tuning in to body signals and energy levels

CLIENT: Sure.

PRACTITIONER: These are a few different directions we could go today. There are many reasons we overeat. One reason is referred to in this first circle, "Paying attention to hunger." Sometimes it's just a matter of eating a meal a little earlier when we aren't quite so ravenous, or adding an afternoon snack. The idea is that if you go into a meal gently hungry, it will be easier to eat slower and to put a preferred amount of food on your plate. Another trigger for overeating is simply not noticing stomach fullness while eating. So another topic we could discuss is slowing the meal down and removing distractions while eating that keep you from paying attention to your meal. We could also talk today about tuning in to your body and simply noticing what foods make you feel good and less lethargic. Or we could talk about food and emotions today. [giving information] Which circle on here, if any, really resonates with you right now? [closed-ended question]

CLIENT: I like the idea of slowing down. I'd say I've got just the right amount of hunger going into a meal, so that's not the problem. The problem is that I'm not really paying attention to my meal while I eat and I'm sometimes going back for seconds when I've really already had enough. I just need to slow down. [change talk—need to change]

PRACTITIONER: Eating slower and checking in with your fullness cue periodically throughout the meal sounds like a good place to start. [reflection of change talk]

CLIENT: I've always been a fast eater. I was the youngest of five children, so I had to eat fast growing up if I wanted seconds.

PRACTITIONER: That eating fast reflex is hardwired and you want to do some rewiring. [reflection—eliciting change talk]

CLIENT: Right. Now it's just me and my husband, so I have no need to eat that fast. [change talk—reasons for change]

PRACTITIONER: This is a good time in your life to make this change because you can do it without worrying about others at the table. [reflection of change talk] Describe that feeling of over-fullness that you're hoping to avoid by slowing down. [open-ended question to evoke change talk]

CLIENT: Ugh, I hate it. I just feel like curling up and taking a nap after dinner. I have no energy to do the dishes.

PRACTITIONER: You feel exhausted. [reflection of change talk] What else? [open-ended question]

CLIENT: I feel bloated. I definitely don't feel like jumping up and doing something after dinner. And then I feel even worse.

PRACTITIONER: There's possibly some guilt and shame mixed up in these overeating experiences. [complex reflection]

CLIENT: And then, sometimes, I eat even more because I feel like I've blown it so I might as well get some more in before I start over again the next day.

PRACTITIONER: This desire for weight loss comes up for you and in a lot of ways makes things worse. [complex reflection]

CLIENT: Yeah, it does!

PRACTITIONER: You're ready to try something different. [reflection that takes a guess at change talk]

CLIENT: Yes, I am. I'm stuck in this vicious cycle. [change talk—activation]

PRACTITIONER: You're ready to break the cycle by slowing down and starting to experience satisfaction while you eat instead of racing to the end. [reflection of change talk]

CLIENT: Yes.

PRACTITIONER: What might you do to remember to slow your pace during your meal? [open-ended question—key question]

In this dialogue, the practitioner uses the focusing process to guide the client toward a specific behavior change within the broad topic of intuitive eating. The practitioner then guides the client into the evoking process with the purpose of eliciting change talk. The script ends with a key question (Chapter 4) to transition the client to the planning process where specific strategies can begin to take shape.

Principle 5: Life-Enhancing Movement

The final HAES principle is centered on supporting "physical activities that allow people of all sizes, abilities, and interests to engage in enjoyable movement, to the degree that they choose."

Dieters often start exercising with the intention of losing weight. Motivation is strong at first, but often wanes as soon as weight plateaus. Furthermore, exercising with a mindset of calories burned can rob the dieter of the joy that is possible with physical activity. When weight loss is the goal, both food and exercise can become drab and unappealing. In a non-diet approach, food and physical activities are selected mindfully based on enjoyment and pleasure. Exercise is no longer viewed as a way to be able to eat more, but as a fun pastime that feels good.

When using a non-diet approach to physical activity, clients are invited to brainstorm the activities they enjoy most. At the same time, clients are exposed to the intrinsic benefits of exercise such as improved sleep, improved body image (regardless of changes in weight), enhanced feelings of physical hunger, and reduced stress, depression, and anxiety. Clients explore their attitudes about exercise and are asked to voice the immediate psychosocial benefits they often experience when they are active. Coaching a client toward mindfulness involves attending to how the body feels while exercising and tuning in to positive and negative attitudes that may arise.

Through tuning clients in to individual body cues, clients learn to pay attention to the various emotional components of eating and activity. Instead of encouraging clients to accept themselves only after the weight has been lost, clients are invited to begin the journey toward a positive body image regardless of size and shape.

As demonstrated throughout this chapter, the spirit of MI can be used as a guide to address your clients' weight concerns. Figure 15.3 summarizes the similarities between the MI spirit and non-diet approaches. Additional resources on adopting non-diet approaches such as the HAES paradigm can be found in Appendix 2, "Additional Resources."

While focusing on weight and body composition may motivate clients to make positive eating and activity changes at first, motivation will be short lived if weight doesn't continue to drop. Sustainable change is achieved when the process of eating and being active is rewarding and enjoyable. Typically, calorie-restricted eating plans and tedious physical activity regimens are far from enjoyable, especially when clients don't see their expectations being met. Helping clients tune in to the moment-to-moment benefits (or intrinsic benefits) of behavior change fuels changes that will last a lifetime.

Spirit of MI	Strategies for addressing clients' weight concerns
Partnership	Treat the client as the expert of his or her body.
Acceptance	Avoid using judgment, shame, or fear as a motivator for behavior change.
Absolute worth	Avoid discrimination, stigmatization, weight bias, and making assumptions.
Accurate empathy	Attempt to see the world through the eyes of clients who experience oppression and stigmatization.
Autonomy support	Give client freedom of choice with food, fitness, and self-care.
Affirmation	Provide affirmations based on changes in attitudes, personal discoveries, and behaviors, not outcomes.
Compassion	Commit to the overall well-being of the client instead of self-gain.
Evocation	Evoke negative aspects of dieting as well as change talk in support of whole-body self-care.

FIGURE 15.3. The spirit of MI as a guide in addressing clients' weight concerns.

Making Referrals

Food and nutrition is a complex topic that easily bleeds into other issues. Popular author on compulsive eating and dieting Geneen Roth (2010) states, "The relationship with food is only a microcosm for your relationship to the rest of your life." Therefore, nutrition counselors often find themselves discussing topics that they aren't formally trained to discuss, such as parenting, communicating with family members, drugs and alcohol, and body image.

The framework that describes this circle of knowledge and skills is known as one's scope of practice. For example, the Scope of Practice in Nutrition and Dietetics encompasses the range of roles, activities, and regulations within which nutrition and dietetics practitioners perform (Academy Quality Management Committee and Scope of Practice Subcommittee of the Quality Management Committee, 2013b). Be sure to investigate both the rigid and flexible boundaries that make up your personal scope of practice. A dietitian's individual scope of practice has flexible boundaries based on personal education, training, credentialing, and demonstrated and documented competence. Boundaries that are more rigid include professional codes, laws, and hospital and clinic policies.

Within every profession, skill sets and level of expertise can expand with training and experience. For example, a new fitness instructor may feel uncomfortable talking about sports nutrition with a client if she received very little training in this area during her education and training programs. However, if the fitness instructor takes a semester-long sports nutrition course as an elective in graduate school, her scope of practice would expand, assuming that tackling these issues wouldn't go against any institutional policies or governing rules and regulations. The scenarios outlined in this book cover a wide scope of practice and are not intended to encourage people to practice outside their lawful business code or code of ethics.

Nutrition and fitness practitioners are at risk for crossing the line into a number of other disciplines, including pharmacy, medicine, addictions counseling, social work, and psychotherapy. One common source of discomfort among nutrition and fitness practitioners is the fuzzy line between behavior change counseling and psychotherapy. The goals of nutrition and fitness counseling and psychotherapy are very different. Counseling performed by a nutritionist or fitness expert typically centers around changing a food or exercise behavior. In psychotherapy, the treatment goals are focused on managing mental illness, mood, emotional healing, and improving relationships.

It is important to remain mindful of your scope of practice. Some signs that you are practicing outside of your scope of practice include:

- A significant amount of the session is on topics unrelated to nutrition and food.
- You have a gut feeling of discomfort or anxiety during a counseling session.
- You get the feeling you may be stepping on the toes of another health care professional.
- You are spending a lot of extra time coordinating care for the client because they could use help "navigating the system."

There are many costs involved with stepping outside of your scope of practice. First, stepping outside of your scope could offend another practitioner. Worse, you could harm a vulnerable client. You can also set yourself up for burnout. It's important to speak up when you notice that a client is struggling with an issue that warrants care from another professional.

REFERRING CLIENTS TO MENTAL HEALTH PROFESSIONALS

Unfortunately, there is some stigma surrounding seeing a mental health professional. Making matters worse, clients are sometimes afraid of talking about their difficult and emotional life trials. Often the nutrition counselor is sought first and seen as less stigmatizing and safer. The client may not be aware of the underlying issues driving her behavioral choices and make an appointment with a nutrition counselor thinking that gaining nutritional knowledge will suffice. Being that there are many complex underlying issues surrounding food and body image, clients' needs are often beyond the scope of a nutrition therapist. Providing a referral to a psychotherapist can be challenging and intimidating to some nutritionists. However, you would never send a broken-down automobile to a motorcycle mechanic, right? It's important to get clients the specialized care they need.

Here are a few signs that your client may benefit from seeing a psychotherapist:

- A heightened concern about body weight or body image, as evidenced by regular weighing; body-bashing language; compensatory behaviors such as vomiting, excessive exercise, diet pill, or laxative abuse; and mood shifts related to weight fluctuations.

- Mention of abuse from others, including physical, sexual, or verbal abuse.
- Marital stress.
- Parenting challenges.
- Loss/grief.
- Emotional states such as sadness, anxiety, depression, hopelessness.
- Suicidal ideation.
- Posttraumatic stress from a previous event.

When making a referral, nutrition therapist and MI expert Molly Kellogg (2009) recommends first providing a reflection or summary that highlights the areas of concern. Next, describe the benefit of meeting with the therapist. In true MI fashion, ask for the client's thoughts on meeting with another professional and finally ask permission before providing names of therapists. These four steps are summarized in Figure A.1 and examples of common referral topics are provided.

When providing referrals, avoid making mental health diagnoses or labeling clients or therapists. For example, which of the following may be better received by a client?

"Your symptoms are consistent with an eating disorder. Would you like to see an eating disorder specialist?"

"You're concerned about how much time you spend thinking about food and weight. Would you like to see someone who specializes in thought patterns surrounding food and body image?"

By avoiding the label of eating disorder, there may be less resistance to seeing the specialist. As the nutrition counselor, you choose whether to make the referral, you control the wording used in communicating this to the client, and you can document that the referral was made. However, you are not in control of whether the client follows through with the referral.

Consistent with the spirit of MI, give the client complete autonomy to follow through with the referral. That does not always mean you must continue to see this client. For example, due to issues with liability and standards of good care, most dietitians refuse to see clients with eating disorders unless the client is also seeing a therapist and physician. While this may seem inconsistent with autonomy, if this policy is clearly communicated to the client, the client still decides whether she will continue with services. You might explain this to the client by stating, "It works best when my clients work with a team that includes a doctor, a therapist, and a dietitian. I want the very best care for you, so I'd be glad to work with you as part of your team, but not alone."

Psychotherapists have specialty areas. Keep a list of therapists in your area

	Example A: Marital conflict	Example B: Eating disorder	Example C: Emotional eating	Example D: Parenting issues
Step 1: Reflect what you hear.	"Last session you shared that you were having a hard time communicating your needs with your husband."	"It sounds like you're thinking about food and body more than you'd like to be. You've given a few examples of how those thoughts have interfered with different areas of your life."	"You shared that anxiety is something you struggle with and you're noticing how stress and anxiety prompt you to eat when you're not necessarily hungry."	"You're concerned that your son's behavior at the dinner table is negatively affecting the eating experience for the entire family. You feel stuck and are hoping to get more ideas about how to set up clear boundaries and rules at the table."
Step 2: Explain how a therapist may be able to help.	"I wonder if it might be helpful to discuss these challenges with someone who specializes in relationships and communication."	"To move forward in reducing these thoughts, many of my clients have found it useful to meet with a counselor who specializes in helping clients navigate this internal battle."	"I know there are a lot of options for managing anxiety. I'm not an expert in that area, but I know others who are."	"You're not alone. Parenting is hard work. There are some well-trained marriage and family therapists in town who have helped other clients of mine figure out solutions for these types of scenarios."
Step 3: Ask what the client thinks.	"What do you think about meeting with someone who could give you some ideas about opening up the lines of communication in your marriage?"	"How do you feel about meeting with a therapist who specializes in food, mood, and body image?"	"What are your thoughts about seeking further assistance in managing your anxiety with someone trained in that area?"	"What are your thoughts on meeting with someone who can help you explore these and other parenting challenges?"
Step 4: Ask permission and provide contact information.	"Would you be interested in some names and phone numbers of some of the experts in our area?"			

FIGURE A1. Four steps to providing a referral.

along with their specialties. Build relationships with these mental health professionals and communicate about referral topics and strategies. Experienced nutrition and fitness practitioners know their place as a member of the health care team. As you gain additional training through continuing education, regularly reassess your individual scope of practice and the scope of practice of professionals in your area. Health care is a team approach and nutrition and fitness professionals, armed with MI, are valuable team members.

Additional Resources

This book serves as a diving board with the hope that you will bounce off and out into the water of nutrition and fitness counseling attempting some of these skills. Just as you can't simply read a book about how to swim and assume you will glide through the water, mastering MI requires practice, supervision, and feedback. Here are some additional resources to assist you in your MI journey.

RESOURCES ON MOTIVATIONAL INTERVIEWING

Books

Miller, W. M., & Rollnick, S. (2013). *Motivational interviewing* (3rd ed.)*: Helping people change.* New York: Guilford Press.—Miller and Rollnick are the developers of MI and this is their third edition. The book provides a thorough overview of MI with sample scripts covering a wide variety of disciplines.

Wagner, C. C., & Ingersoll, K. S. (2012). *Motivational interviewing in groups.* New York: Guilford Press.—An excellent resource for those who wish to apply MI skills when facilitating group classes and group support programs.

Rosengren, D. B. (2009). *Building motivational interviewing skills: A practitioner workbook.* New York: Guilford Press.—This workbook includes activities to facilitate practicing MI skills.

Rollnick, S., Miller, W. M., & Butler, C. C. (2007). *Motivational interviewing in health care: Helping patients change behavior.* New York: Guilford Press.— The authors provide an overview of MI with scripts that are specific to the health professions.

Naar-King, S., & Suarez, M. (2010). *Motivational interviewing with adolescents and young adults.* New York: Guilford Press.—This book provides suggestions for using MI from a developmentally informed perspective and addresses many issues specific to adolescents and young adults such as sexual risk taking, substance abuse, and eating disorders.

Website

www.motivationalinterviewing.org—The Motivational Interviewing Network of Trainers (MINT) is an international, cross-disciplinary organization that was started in 1997 by a small group of trainers educated by MI founders William R. Miller and Stephen Rollnick. There are many useful resources on this website, including information about how to become a member of MINT.

RESOURCES FOR NUTRITION COUNSELING

Molly Kellogg, RD, LCSW

Molly Kellogg, a psychotherapist and nutrition therapist, offers extensive materials on MI and nutrition counseling, all of which can be accessed on her website: *www.mollykellogg.com*. There you will find 50 free nutrition counseling tips. She also offers trainings all over the country and supervision services. Here are a few of her products:

Counseling tips for nutrition therapists: Practice workbook series (Vols. 1–3).

Steps to counseling excellence: A program for practicing nutrition professionals.

Book

Constance, A., & Sauter, C. (2011). *Inspiring and supporting behavior change: A food and nutrition professional's counseling guide.* Chicago: American Dietetic Association.—While there are other books on nutrition counseling, most provide very little on MI. However, this book includes several chapters that address these concepts.

RESOURCES ON FITNESS COUNSELING

There are currently no known books on exercise counseling that specifically address MI. However, the following websites may be helpful:

www.acsm.org—The website of the American College of Sports Medicine (ACSM), the primary sports medicine and exercise science organization in the world.

http://exerciseismedicine.org/index.php—The website of Exercise is Medicine®, a global health initiative managed by ACSM, that provides resources for health care providers to include physical activity when designing treatment plans for patients. The following toolkit is for dietitians who are addressing physical activity during counseling sessions: *www.exerciseismedicine.org/assets/page_documents/WM%20EIM%20Toolkit%202013%20FINAL.pdf.*

www.appliedsportpsych.org—The website of the Association for Applied Sport and Exercise Psychology (AASP), a sport and exercise psychology professional organization. They have health and fitness resources that are useful for exercise counseling: *www.appliedsportpsych.org/resource-center/health-fitness-resources*.

RESOURCES ON ADDRESSING WEIGHT AND BODY IMAGE CONCERNS WITH CLIENTS

Books

Glovsky, E. (Ed.). (2014). *Wellness, not weight: Health at every size and motivational interviewing.* San Diego: Cognella.—This book includes a brief overview of MI and a compilation of chapters written by authors with expertise in the weight-neutral, HAES paradigm. Topics addressed include the latest research on weight and health, mindful eating, eating competence, sports nutrition, food and feelings, eating disorders, and communicating a non-diet approach to clients using MI.

Matz, J., & Frankl, E. (2014). *Beyond a shadow of a diet: The therapist's guide to treating compulsive eating.* New York: Brunner-Routledge.—This book was written for practitioners who work with clients struggling with binge-eating disorder, compulsive eating, or emotional overeating. The authors demonstrate how to incorporate the HAES paradigm into counseling sessions and also address topics such as the clinician's own attitudes toward dieting and weight; cultural, ethical, and social justice issues; the neuroscience of mindfulness; weight stigma; and promoting wellness for children of all sizes.

Willer, F. (2013). *The non-diet approach guidebook for dietitians.* Raleigh, NC: Lulu Press.—This book explains the non-diet approach and provides strategies for incorporating these approaches into nutrition and dietetics, including strategies for medical charting and following the Nutrition Care Process.

Adams, L., & Willer, F. (2014). *The non-diet approach guidebook for psychologists and counsellors.* Lulu Press.—This book explains the non-diet approach and provides strategies for incorporating these approaches into a psychological counseling practice.

Websites

www.sizediversityandhealth.org—The website of the Association for Size Diversity and Health, an international professional organization composed of members committed to the HAES principles. This website includes the HAES principles, resources, and webinars.

www.amIhungry.com—The website of the Am I Hungry® company, run by a physician, Dr. Michelle May. There are many resources on mindful eating for both professionals and clients, including books, trainings for professionals, and retreats for clients.

www.intuitiveeating.com—A website developed by the authors of the book *Intuitive Eating*, Evelyn Tribole, MS, RD, and Elyse Resch, MS, RD, FADA. There are resources for clients and practitioners, including a free intuitive eating online community.

www.lindabacon.org—The homepage of HAES author and advocate Dr. Linda Bacon. She offers books and resources for clients and practitioners.

www.haescommunity.org—A website developed by Dr. Linda Bacon to create community among HAES advocates. There are registries for finding HAES practitioners, resource lists, and pledges.

www.haescurriculum.com—A website that provides free materials for teaching HAES concepts. This curriculum was developed as a joint venture by the Association for Size Diversity and Health, the National Association for the Advancement of Fat Acceptance, and the Society for Nutrition Education and Behavior. There are PowerPoints that can be downloaded, prerecorded lectures about HAES concepts for streaming and assignment, and reading lists for university professors who wish to incorporate these concepts into course curricula.

References

Academy Quality Management Committee & Scope of Practice Subcommittee of the Quality Management Committee. (2013a). Academy of Nutrition and Dietetics: Scope of Practice in Nutrition and Dietetics. *Journal of the Academy of Nutrition and Dietetics, 113*(6, Suppl.), S11–S16.

Academy Quality Management Committee & Scope of Practice Subcommittee of the Quality Management Committee. (2013b). Academy of Nutrition and Dietetics: Revised 2012 Standards of Practice in Nutrition Care and Standards of Professional Performance for Registered Dietitians. *Journal of the Academy of Nutrition and Dietetics, 113*(6, Suppl. 2), S29–S45.

Amy, N. K., Aalborg A., Lyons P., & Keranen L. (2006). Barriers to routine gynecological cancer screening for white and African-American obese women. *International Journal of Obesity, 30*(1), 147–155.

Armstrong, M. J., Mottershead, T. A., Ronksley, P. E., Sigal, R. J., Campbell, T. S., & Hemmelgarn, B. R. (2011). Motivational interviewing to improve weight loss in overweight and/or obese patients: A systematic review and meta-analysis of randomized controlled trials. *Obesity Reviews, 12*(9), 709–723.

Association for Size Diversity and Health. (2014). Health At Every Size principles. Retrieved January 3, 2015, from *www.sizediversityandhealth.org/content.asp?d=152*.

Bacon, L., & Aphramor, L. (2011). Weight science: Evaluating the evidence for a paradigm shift. *Nutrition Journal, 10*, 69.

Bacon, L., Keim, N., Van Loan, M., Derricote, M., Gale, B., Kazaks, A., et al. (2002). Evaluating a "non-diet" wellness intervention for improvement of metabolic fitness, psychological well-being and eating and activity behaviors. *International Journal of Obesity, 26*, 854–865.

Bacon, L., Stern, J. S., Van Loan, M. D., & Keim, N. L. (2005). Size acceptance and intuitive eating improve health for obese, female chronic dieters. *Journal of the American Dietetic Association, 105*, 929–936.

Barnett, E., Moyers, T. B., Sussman, S., Smith, C., Rohrbach, L. A., Sun, P., et al. (2014). From counselor skill to decreased marijuana use: Does change talk matter? *Journal of Substance Abuse Treatment, 46*(4), 498–505.

Barry, V. W., Beets, M. W., Durstine, J. L., Liu, J., & Blair, S. N. (2014). Fitness vs. fatness on all-cause mortality: A meta-analysis. *Progress in Cardiovascular Diseases, 56*, 382–390.

Bean, M. K., Powell, P., Quinoy, A., Ingersoll, K., Wickham, E. P., & Mazzeo, S. E. (2015). Motivational interviewing targeting diet and physical activity improves adherence to paediatric obesity treatment: Results from the MI values randomized controlled trial. *Pediatric Obesity, 10*, 118–125.

Beck, A. T. (2005). The current state of cognitive therapy: A 40-year retrospective. *Archives of General Psychiatry, 62*, 953–959.

Brodie, D. A., Inour, A., & Shaw, D. G. (2006). Motivational interviewing to change quality of life for people with chronic heart failure: A randomized controlled trial. *International Journal of Nursing Studies, 45*, 489–500.

Campbell, K., & Crawford, D. (2000). Management of obesity: Attitudes and practices of Australian dietitians. *International Journal of Obesity, 24*, 701–710.

Campbell, M. K., Carr, C., DeVellis, B., Switer, B., Biddle, A., Amamo, M. A., et al. (2009). A randomized trial of tailoring and motivational interviewing to promote fruit and vegetable consumption for cancer prevention and control. *Annals of Behavioral Medicine, 38*, 71–85.

Centers for Disease Control and Prevention. (2014). Facts about physical activity. Retrieved May 21, 2014, from *www.cdc.gov/physicalactivity/data/facts.html.*

Chinn, D. J., White, M., Harland, J., Drinkwater, C., & Raybould, S. (1999). Barriers to physical activity and socioeconomic position: Implications for health promotion. *Journal of Epidemiology in Community Health, 53*, 191–192.

Christison, A. L., Daley, B. M., Asche, C. V., Ren, J., Aldag, J. C., Ariza, A. J., et al. (2014). Pairing motivational interviewing with a nutrition and physical activity assessment and counseling tool in pediatric clinical practice: A pilot study. *Childhood Obesity. 10*(5), 1–10.

Clifford, D., Ozier, A., Bundros, J., Moore, J., Kreiser, A., & Neyman Morris, M. (2015). Impact of non-diet approaches on attitudes, behaviors, and health outcomes: A systematic review. *Journal of Nutrition Education and Behavior, 47*(2), 143–155.

Dansinger, M. L., Gleason, J. A., Griffith, J. L., Selker, H. P., & Schaefer, E. J. (2005). Comparison of the Atkins, Ornish, Weight Watchers, and Zone diets for weight loss and heart disease risk reduction. *Journal of the American Medical Association, 293*, 43–53.

Dansinger, M. L., Tatsioni, A., Wong, J. B., Chung, M., & Balk, E. M. (2007). Meta-analysis: The effect of dietary counseling for weight loss. *Annals of Internal Medicine, 147*, 41–50.

Deci, E. L., & Cascio, W. F. (1972). *Changes in intrinsic motivation as a function of negative feedback and threats.* Paper presented at the 43rd annual meeting of the Eastern Psychological Association, Boston, MA.

Deci, E. L., Koestner, R., & Ryan, R. M. (1999). A meta-analytic review of experiments examining the effects of extrinsic rewards on intrinsic motivation. *Psychological Bulletin, 125*, 627–668.

Deci, E. L., & Ryan, R. M. (2008). Facilitating optimal motivation and psychological well-being across life's domains. *Canadian Psychology, 49*, 14–23.

Diener, E., & Seligman, M. E. P. (2004). Beyond money: Toward an economy of well-being. *Psychological Science in the Public Interest, 5*, 1–31.

Dishman, R. K. (1991). Increasing and maintaining exercise and physical activity. *Behaviour Therapy, 22*, 345–378.

Eisenberg, M. E., Neumark-Sztainer, D., & Story, M. (2003). Associations of weight-based teasing and emotional well-being among adolescents. *Archives of Pediatric and Adolescent Medicine, 157*(8), 733–738.

Epstein, L. H., Temple, J. L., Roemmich, J. N., & Bouton, M. E. (2009). Habituation as a determinant of human food intake. *Psychology Review, 116*, 384–407.

Fang, J., Wylie-Rosett, J., Cohen, H. W., Kaplan, R. C., & Alderman, M. H. (2003). Exercise, body mass index, caloric intake, and cardiovascular mortality. *American Journal of Preventative Medicine, 4*, 283–289.

Flegal, K. M., Kit, B. K., Orpana, H., & Graubard, B. I. (2013). Association of all-cause mortality with overweight and obesity using standard body mass index categories: A systematic review and meta-analysis. *Journal of the American Medical Association, 309*(1), 71–82.

Frey, A. J., Cloud, R. N., Lee, J., Small, J. W., Seeley, J. R., Feil, E. G., et al. (2011). The promise of motivational interviewing in school mental health. *School Mental Health, 3*(1), 1–12.

Garber, C. E., Blissmer, B., Deschenes, M. R., Franklin, B., Lamonte, M. J., Lee, I. M., et al. (2011). Quantity and quality of exercise for developing and maintaining cardiorespiratory, musculoskeletal, and neuromotor fitness in apparently health adults: Guidance for prescribing exercise. *Medicine and Science in Sports and Exercise, 43*(7), 1334–1359.

Gaume, J., Bertholet, N., Faouzi, M., Gmel, G., & Daeppen, J. B. (2013). Does change talk during brief motivational interventions with young men predict change in alcohol use? *Journal of Substance Abuse Treatment, 44*(2), 177–185.

Glovsky, E. (2012). Training with Dr. Ellen: Training and consultation in motivational interviewing. Retrieved November 26, 2012, from *http://trainingwithdrellen.com*.

Heckman, C. J., Egleston, B. L., & Hofmann, M. T. (2010). Efficacy of motivational interviewing for smoking cessation: A systematic review and meta-analysis. *Tobacco Control, 19*(5), 410–416.

Hollis, J. L., Williams, L. T., Collins, C. E., & Morgan, P. J. (2014). Does motivational interviewing align with international scope of practice, professional competency standards, and best practice guidelines in dietetics practice? *Journal of the Academy for Nutrition and Dietetics 115*, 676–687.

Johnston, C. A. (2012). The impact of weight-based discrimination in the health care setting. *American Journal of Lifestyle Medicine, 6*, 452–454.

Kellogg, M. (2009). *Counseling tips for nutrition therapists: Practice workbook* (Vol. 2). Philadelphia: Kg Press.

Kowalski, P. (2010). *A manual for exercise adherence consulting with college students*. Unpublished master's thesis, California State University, Chico, CA.

Lacey, K., & Pritchett, E. (2003). Nutrition Care Process and Model: ADA adopts road map to quality care and outcomes management. *Journal of the American Dietetic Association, 103*(8), 1061–1072.

Landry, J. B., & Solmon, M. A. (2004). African American women's self-determination across the stages for change for exercise. *Journal of Sport and Exercise Psychology, 26,* 257–469.

Lantz, P. M., Golberstein, E., House, J. S., & Morenoff, J. (2010). Socioeconomic and behavioral risk factors for mortality in a national 19-year prospective study of U.S. adults. *Social Science and Medicine, 70*(10), 1558–1566.

Latner, J. D., Durso, L. E., & Mond, J. M. (2013). Health and health-related quality of life among treatment-seeking overweight and obese adults: Associations with internalized weight bias. *Journal of Eating Disorders, 1,* 3.

Lundahl, B., Moleni, T., Burke, B. L., Butters, R., Tollefson, D., Butler, C., et al. (2013). Motivational interviewing in medical care settings: A systematic review and meta-analysis of randomized controlled trials. *Patient Education and Counseling, 93*(2), 157–168.

MacDonnell, K., Brogan, K., Naar-King, S., Ellis, D., & Marshall, S. (2012). A pilot study of motivational interviewing targeting weight-related behaviors in overweight or obese African American adolescents. *Journal of Adolescent Health, 50*(2), 201–203.

MacLean, P. S., Bergoulgnan, M. C., Cornier, M., & Jackman, M. R. (2011). Biology's response to dieting: The impetus for weight regain. *American Journal of Physiology–Regulatory, Integrative and Comparative Physiology, 301,* R581–R600.

Mahle Lutter, J., Rex, J., Hawkes, C., & Bucaccio, P. (1999). Incentives and barriers to physical activity for working women. *American Journal of Health Promotion, 13*(4), 215–218.

Mann, T., Tomiyama, J., Westling, E., Lew, A. M., Samuels, B., & Chatman, J. (2007). Medicare's search for effective obesity treatments. *American Psychologist, 62*(3), 220–233.

Marketdata Enterprises, Inc. (2011). *The U.S. weight loss and diet control market.* Rockville, MD: Author.

Mathieu, J. (2009). What should you know about mindful and intuitive eating? *Journal of the American Dietetic Association, 109*(12), 1982.

McMurran, M. (2009). Motivational interviewing with offenders: A systematic review. *Legal and Criminological Psychology, 14*(1), 83–100.

Miller, W. R. (Ed.). (2004). *Combined behavioral intervention manual: A clinical research guide for therapists treating people with alcohol abuse and dependence* (Vol. 1). Bethesda, MD: National Institute on Alcohol Abuse and Alcoholism.

Miller, S. T., Oates, V. J., Brooks, M. A., Shintani, A., Gebretsadik, T., & Jenkins, D. M. (2014). Preliminary efficacy of group medical nutrition therapy and motivational interviewing among obese African American women with type 2 diabetes: A pilot study. *Journal of Obesity, 2014.*

Miller, W. R., & Rollnick, S. (1991). *Motivational interviewing: Preparing people to change.* New York: Guilford Press.

Miller, W. R., & Rollnick, S. (2002). *Motivational interviewing: Preparing people for change* (2nd ed.). New York: Guilford Press.

Miller, W. R., & Rollnick, S. (2013). *Motivational interviewing: Helping people change* (3rd ed.). New York: Guilford Press.

Miller, W. R., & Rose, G. S. (2009). Toward a theory of motivational interviewing. *American Psychologist, 64*(6), 527–537.

Neumark-Sztainer, D. R., Friend, S. E., Flattum, C. F., Hannan, P. J., Story, M., Bauer, K. W., et al. (2010). New Moves—preventing weight-related problems in adolescent girls: A group randomized study. *American Journal of Preventative Medicine, 39,* 421–432.

Neumark-Sztainer, D. [R.], Wall, M., Guo, J., Story, M., Haines, J., & Eisenberg, M. (2006). Obesity, disordered eating, and eating disorders in a longitudinal study of adolescents: How do dieters fare 5 years later? *Journal of the American Dietetic Association, 106,* 559–568.

Norcross, J. C., Mrykalo, M. S., & Blagys, M. D. (2002). Auld Lang Syne: Success predictors, change processes, and self-reported outcomes of New Year's resolvers and nonresolvers. *Journal of Clinical Psychology, 58*(4), 397–405.

Plant, R., & Ryan, R. M. (1985). Intrinsic motivation and the effects of self-consciousness, self-awareness, and ego-involvement: An investigation of internally controlling styles. *Journal of Personality, 53,* 435–449.

Polivy, J., Coleman, J., & Herman, C. P. (2005). The effect of deprivation on food cravings and eating behavior in restrained and unrestrained eaters. *International Journal of Eating Disorders, 38,* 301–309.

Polivy, J., & Herman, C. P. (1999). Effects of resolving to diet on restrained and unrestrained eaters: The "false hope syndrome." *International Journal of Eating Disorders, 26,* 434–447.

Polivy, J., & Herman, C. P. (2000). The false-hope syndrome: Unfulfilled expectations of self change. *Current Directions in Psychological Science, 9*(4), 128–131.

Prichard, M., & Tiggemann, M. (2008). An examination of pre-wedding body image concerns in brides and bridesmaids. *Body Image, 5*(4), 395–398.

Prochaska, J. O., & DiClemente, C. C. (1984). *The transtheoretical approach: Crossing traditional boundaries of therapy.* Homewood, IL: Dow/Jones Irwin.

Puhl, R. M., & Brownell, K. D. (2006). Confronting and coping with weight stigma: An investigation of overweight and obese adults. *Obesity, 14*(10), 1802–1815.

Ramos Salas, X. (2015). The ineffectiveness and unintended consequences of the public health war on obesity. *Canadian Journal of Public Health, 106*(2), 79–81.

Richins, M. (1991). Social comparison and idealized images of advertising. *Journal of Consumer Research, 18,* 71–83.

Rogers, C. (1995). What understanding and acceptance mean to me. *Journal of Humanistic Psychology, 35,* 7–22.

Rollnick, S., Miller, W. R., & Butler, C. C. (2008). *Motivational interviewing in health care.* New York: Guilford Press.

Rosen, J. C., Reiter, J., & Orosan, P. (1995). Cognitive-behavioral body image therapy for body dysmorphic disorder. *Journal of Consulting and Clinical Psychology, 63*(2), 263–269.

Rosengren, D. B. (2009). *Building motivational interviewing skills: A practitioner workbook.* New York: Guilford Press.

Roth, G. (2010). *Women, food, and God: An unexpected path to almost everything.* New York: Scribner.

Ryan, R. M., & Deci, E. L. (2000). Intrinsic and extrinsic motivations: Classic definitions and new directions. *Contemporary Educational Psychology, 25*, 54–67.

Satter, E. (2008). *Secrets of feeding a healthy family: How to eat, how to raise good eaters, how to cook.* Madison, WI: Kelcy Press.

Schaefer, J. T., & Magnuson, A. B. (2014). A review of interventions that promote eating by internal cues. *Journal of the Academy of Nutrition and Dietetics, 114*(5), 734–760.

Sikorski, C., Luppa, M., Kaiser, M., Glaesmer, H., Schomerus, G., Konig, H. H., et al. (2011). The stigma of obesity in the general public and its implications for public health: A systematic review. *BMC Public Health, 11*, 661.

Snetselaar, L. (2008). *Nutrition counseling skills for the nutrition care process* (4th ed.). Sudbury, MA: Jones & Bartlett.

Spoor, S., Stice, E., Bekker, M., Van Strien, T., Croon, M. A., & Van Heck, G. L. (2006). Relations between dietary restraint, depressive symptoms and binge eating: A longitudinal study. *International Journal of Eating Disorders, 39*, 700–707.

Steinhardt, M., Bezner, J., & Adams, T. (1999). Outcomes of a traditional weight control program and a nondiet alternative: A one-year comparison. *Journal of Psychology, 133*, 495–513.

Stice, E., Cameron, R. P., Killen, J. D., Hayward, C., & Taylor, C. B. (1999). Naturalistic weight-reduction efforts prospectively predict growth in relative weight and onset of obesity among female adolescents. *Journal of Consulting and Clinical Psychology, 67*, 967–974.

Stott, N., Rollnick, S., Rees, M., & Pill, R. (1995). Innovation in clinical method: Diabetes care and negotiating skills. *Family Practice, 12*(4), 413–418.

Sumithran, P., & Proietto, J. (2013). The defence of body weight: A physiological basis for weight regain after weight loss. *Clinical Science, 124*, 231–241.

Sustin, A. R., & Terracciano, A. (2014). Perceived weight discrimination and obesity. *PLoS ONE, 8*(7), e70048.

Swift, J. A., Hanlon, S., El-Redy, L., Puhl, R. M., & Glazebrook, C. (2012). Weight bias among UK trainee dietitians, doctors, nurses and nutritionists. *Journal of Human Nutrition and Dietetics, 26*(4), 395–402.

Thomas, S. L., Lewis, S., Hyde, J., Castle, D., & Komesaroff, P. (2010). The solution needs to be complex: Obese adults' attitudes about the effectiveness of individual and population based interventions for obesity. *BMC Public Health, 10*, 420.

Tomiyama, A. J. (2014). Weight stigma is stressful: A review of evidence for the Cyclic Obesity/Weight-Based Stigma model. *Appetite, 82*, 8–15.

Tomiyama, A. J., Ahlstrom, B., & Mann, T. (2013). Long-term effects of dieting: Is weight loss related to health? *Social and Personality Psychology Compass, 7*(12), 861–877.

Tribole, E., & Resch, E. (2012). *Intuitive eating* (3rd ed.). New York: St. Martin's Griffin.

Tylka, T. L., Annunziato, R. A., Burgard, D., Danielsdottir, S., Shuman, E., Davis, C., et al. (2014). The weight-inclusive versus weight-normative approach to health: Evaluating the evidence for prioritizing well-being over weight loss. *Journal of Obesity, 2014*, 1–18.

Urbszat, D., Herman, C. P., & Polivy, J. (2002). Eat, drink, and be merry, for tomorrow we diet: Effects of anticipated deprivation on food intake in restrained and unrestrained eaters. *Journal of Abnormal Psychology, 111*(2), 396–401.

Vader, A. M., Walters, S. T., Prabhu, G. C., Houck, J. M., & Field, C. A. (2010). The language of motivational interviewing and feedback: Counselor language, client language, and client drinking outcomes. *Psychology of Addictive Behaviors, 24*(2), 190–197.

Vallerand, R. J., & Reid, G. (1984). On the causal effects of perceived competence on intrinsic motivation: A test of cognitive evaluation theory. *Journal of Sport Psychology, 6*, 94–102.

Van Keulen, H. M., Mesters, I., Ausems, M., van Breukelen, G., Campbell, M., Resnicow, K., et al. (2011). Tailored print communication and motivational interviewing are equally successful in improving multiple lifestyle behaviors in a randomized controlled trial. *Annals of Behavioral Medicine, 41*, 104–118.

VanWormer, J. J., & Boucher, J. L. (2004). Motivational interviewing and diet modification: A review of the evidence. *The Diabetes Educator, 30*, 404–419.

Vartanian, L. R., & Novak, S. A. (2011). Internalized societal attitudes moderate the impact of weight stigma on weight stigma on avoidance of exercise. *Obesity, 19*(4), 757–762.

Vartanian, L. R., & Shaprow, J. G. (2008). Effects of weight stigma on exercise motivation and behavior: A preliminary investigation among college-aged females. *Journal of Health Psychology, 13*(1), 131–138.

Washington, R. L. (2011). Childhood obesity: Issues of weight bias. *Preventing Chronic Disease, 8*(5), A94.

West, D. S., DiLillo, V., Bursac, Z., Gore, S. A., & Greene, P. G. (2007). Motivational interviewing improves weight loss in women with type 2 diabetes. *Diabetes Care, 30*, 1081–1087.

Witte, K., & Allen, M. (2000). A meta-analysis of fear appeals: Implications for effective public health campaigns. *Health Education and Behavior, 27*(5), 591–615.

Index

Note. f following a page number indicates a figure.